CPH Exam

Quick Reference Review

Larry Holmes, Jr., PhD, DrPH
Clinical Epidemiologist
Alfred I. duPont Hospital for Children
Wilmington, Delaware

JONES AND BARTLETT PUBLISHERS
Sudbury, Massachusetts
BOSTON TORONTO LONDON SINGAPORE

World Headquarters
Jones and Bartlett Publishers
40 Tall Pine Drive
Sudbury, MA 01776
978-443-5000
info@jbpub.com
www.jbpub.com

Jones and Bartlett Publishers
Canada
6339 Ormindale Way
Mississauga, Ontario L5V 1J2
Canada

Jones and Bartlett Publishers
International
Barb House, Barb Mews
London W6 7PA
United Kingdom

Jones and Bartlett's books and products are available through most bookstores and online booksellers. To contact Jones and Bartlett Publishers directly, call 800-832-0034, fax 978-443-8000, or visit our website www.jbpub.com.

Substantial discounts on bulk quantities of Jones and Bartlett's publications are available to corporations, professional associations, and other qualified organizations. For details and specific discount information, contact the special sales department at Jones and Bartlett via the above contact information or send an email to specialsales@jbpub.com.

Production Credits
Publisher: Michael Brown
Production Director: Amy Rose
Associate Editor: Katey Birtcher
Production Editor: Tracey Chapman
Marketing Manager: Sophie Fleck
Manufacturing and Inventory Control Supervisor: Amy Bacus
Composition: Arlene Apone
Cover Design: Brian Moore
Cover Image: © Daniela Illing/ShutterStock, Inc.
Printing and Binding: Malloy, Incorporated
Cover Printing: Malloy, Incorporated

Library of Congress Cataloging-in-Publication Data
Holmes, Larry, 1960-
CPH exam quick reference review / Larry Holmes.
p. ; cm.
Includes bibliographical references and index.
ISBN-13: 978-0-7637-6129-5 (pbk.)
ISBN-10: 0-7637-6129-X (pbk.)
1. Public health--Examinations, questions, etc. I. Title. II. Title: Certification in public health exam quick reference review.
[DNLM: 1. Public Health--Problems and Exercises. WA 18.2 H751c 2009]
RA430.H65 2009
362.1076--dc22
2008006664

6048

Printed in the United States of America
12 11 10 09 08 10 9 8 7 6 5 4 3 2 1

DEDICATION

To the memory of Mrs. Elizabeth Kolwes of Brenham, Texas, whose life and dedication to her children, grandchildren, and great-grandchildren reflect a true leadership in public health, thanks to her perpetual application of the fundamental principles of family/economic support system in enabling her family and community health status.

To those who labored and continue to labor for the elimination of education, gender, age, social class, income, and racial/ethnic disparities in health.

CONTENTS

FOREWORD

Public health, the science and art of disease prevention and health promotion, remains significant in the advances of medical and health sciences in ameliorating the health of the population. The contributions of public health to the health of the U.S. population has been remarkable in the 21st century, and it continues to be so as public health confronts emerging challenges due to the aging U.S. population, climate changes, global warming, bioterrorism, and emerging pathogenic microbes. Remarkably, the epidemiologic transition from infectious diseases as the leading cause of mortality in 1900s to chronic diseases today came as a result of persistent immunization and the reduction in vaccine-preventable diseases, thanks to public health efforts. Illustratively, public health achievements in the 21st century are viewed in light of their contributions to motor vehicle safety, safer workplaces, infectious disease control, decline in coronary artery disease and stroke mortality, safer and healthier food, healthier mothers and babies, family planning, fluorination of drinking water, vaccination, and recognition of tobacco as a health hazard.

The scope of public health is broad and reflects what we, as a society, do collectively to ensure the conditions necessary for people to remain healthy. Within this scope, the framework for public health performance recommends the collaboration between governmental agencies (federal, state, and local), public and private sectors, and the communities. The Institute of Medicine, in its 1988 response to "public health in disarray," clearly described the core functions of public health as: (1) assessment, (2) policy development, and (3) assurance. The process upon which public health carries these out requires the integration of its core functions into the essential public health services, namely, (1) health services monitoring and identification of community health needs; (2) diagnoses and investigation of health problems and health hazards in the community; (3) informing, educating, and empowering people about health issues; (4) mobilizing community partnerships to identify and solve health problems; (5) enforcing laws and regulations that protect and ensure safety; (6) linking people with needed personal health services and ensuring the provision of health care when otherwise unavailable; (7) ensuring a competent public health and personal healthcare workforce; (8) evaluating effectiveness, accessibility, and quality of personal and population-based health services; and (9) researching new insights and innovative solutions to health problems.

The training of public health professionals to address the essential public health services requires a curriculum that integrates the core functions of public health into the core disciplines of public health, mainly (1) epidemiology, (2) biostatistics, (3) behavioral and social sciences, (4) environmental sciences, and (5) management and policy sciences. The knowledge of these areas and the application of cross-cutting core competencies (such as communication and informatics, diversity and culture, animal control, public health biology and pathology, professionalism, programs planning, and systems thinking) serve to provide the graduates of public health programs with the preparation (knowledge and skills) needed to succeed in this field today.

The author and the contributors of this text, the *CPH Exam Quick Reference Review*, have presented—in a simplified and concise manner—the introduction to public health as public health principles and practice, which is rarely presented in graduate programs, and have discussed the mission, goal, core functions, history, and challenges of public health. Whereas graduates of public health tend to focus on a set module or discipline, in spite of our recommendation of the broad knowledge of the public health core disciplines, this review has made it possible for graduates and potential graduates of public health to acquire competency in these core areas. This book is intended to prepare graduates of public health for an important examination that will bring collegiality and credibility to this profession. I hope that this review will point readers in a direction that will stimulate their appetite to learn more about the assessment of health issues in the population, about making sense of data, about the role of behavior in health, about the impact of environment on health, and about policy development in the management of public health services. The practice test as presented here serves to introduce readers and candidates of this examination to proper test-taking skills. Therefore, as you attempt these questions, note that your ability to interpret similar questions will enhance your success in the upcoming examination. My hope is that this review will enhance rather than disable your success in the examination. If you believe that all books are perspectives, then no book, no matter the volume, will be able to present all the subject matter of any given field. Therefore, increase your score by using these materials in combination with similar sources of information judged to be relevant in public health examination review.

James Harlan Steele, DVM, MPH
Retired U.S. Assistant Surgeon General
Professor Emeritus, University of Texas
Health Sciences Center at Houston
School of Public Health, Houston, Texas

ACKNOWLEDGMENTS

Public health is an interdisciplinary science, requiring many subspecialties in its approach to disease prevention and health promotion. This review would never have been prepared without contributions from my colleagues from the various disciplines that sustain essential public health functions and research infrastructures. Whereas I do assume partial credit for preparing this review to assist candidates preparing for the National Public Health Certification Examination, any errors originating from the use of this material are absolutely mine.

The idea to write this book stems from the absence of materials available to aid in the preparation for the first National Public Health Certification Examination in the United States during summer 2008. A certification examination in this perspective is challenging—and will remain so, pending transition in the presentation of public health core areas and their core competencies at the graduate level. Schools of public health had traditionally prepared students to focus on their module or discipline with very little exposure to mastery in the five core disciplines: epidemiology, biostatistics, behavioral and social sciences, environmental sciences, and management and policy sciences. Realistically, graduate programs are designed to create a focus, thus gearing toward specialized knowledge. However, a broad knowledge of these core disciplines requires not only introductory courses in these core areas but some level of formation and application of these concepts in the real world. With this gap in mind, this review has made it possible for graduates of public health programs to acquire some mastery in these core areas and the cross-cutting areas (communications and informatics, diversity and culture, leadership, public health biology, professionalism, programs planning, and systems thinking).

Many sources of information were consulted during the gestational period of this review. I am very grateful to all authors whose works we have consulted prior to the preparation of this review. I sincerely appreciate the knowledge and information gained from your intense and meaningful contributions to the field of public health. However, if you feel you have not been adequately acknowledged, I am willing to do so at the first opportunity.

I am indebted to my colleagues at the Texas Medical Center, who provided instant assistance when required to assemble research materials for the many sections in this book that required extra-intense review. Jennifer Thompson, MS, MA, MPH, and Priya Veherdra, MS, MPH, assisted in making sure that the Environmental Sciences in Public Health chapter of this book covered the basics of the environmental sciences enough to provide a broad knowledge of this discipline for public health graduates, regardless of their module, discipline, or concentration. There are others who provided similar assistance. I acknowledge, with thanks, your contributions.

I owe the basic sciences of public health chapters to the experience gained from teaching graduate students in Texas and medical students in the Caribbean over the many years of my teaching career. Because teaching is a learning experience, I have learned by teaching epidemiology and biostatistics in these settings. I hope this experience reflects the information provided in these two chapters.

I am indebted to my parents for never asking me not to ask them "Why?" I am grateful to Jenni, Maddy, MacKenzie, and Landon, and their grandparents, Dalton and Sue, for their patience and unconditional acceptance even when I avoided contact with them and turned to the computer in order to complete a sentence or section of this review.

Public health is not an exact science. We have consulted with sources of information judged to be valid during the period of the preparation of this review. However, information presented today is subject to change as new information becomes available tomorrow. Therefore, readers are required to consult with similar sources for the confirmation of information provided here.

ABOUT THE AUTHOR

Larry Holmes, Jr., PhD, DrPH has over nine years of experience as a reviewer of the United Sates Medical Licensing Examination (USMLE) questions (1994–2003). During this period, he taught the quantitative medicine (epidemiology, biostatistics) among other courses, and was responsible for both the summative and formative examination preparation materials for the medical schools in the Caribbean.

At the International University of the Health Sciences (IUHS) in St. Kitts, Holmes directed the assessment for the basic medical sciences and clinical correlates and managed over 18 thousand questions in the examination bank. He was responsible for preparing the summative examination of 350 questions for every organ-system in the USMLE learning objectives, and these examinations were offered every three months at IUHS. Holmes also wrote review questions for immunology and infectious diseases, quantitative medicine (epidemiology and biostatistics), preventive medicine, behavioral sciences, geriatrics, and pharmacology.

Dr. Holmes is currently a Clinical Epidemiologist at the Alfred I. duPont Hospital for Children in Wilmington, Delaware where he directs the clinical research methodology (modern epidemiology and biostatistics) research and education program. He is a published primary or senior author in many peer reviewed scientific journals, a reviewer for scientific journals including Military Medicine and AIDS Care and a member of the American College of Epidemiology.

CONTRIBUTORS TO *CPH EXAM QUICK REFERENCE REVIEW*

Foreword

James H. Steele, DVM, MPH
Retired U.S. Assistant Surgeon General
Professor Emeritus
University of Texas, School of Public Health
Houston, Texas

Author

Larry Holmes, Jr., PhD, DrPH
Clinical Epidemiologist
Alfred I. duPont Hospital for Children
Wilmington, Delaware

Contributors

Doriel D. Ward, PhD, MPH
Health Policy and Management Sciences and Behavioral Sciences
University of Texas, MD Anderson Cancer Center
Houston, Texas

Jennifer Thompson, MS, MA, MPH
Environmental Sciences
Harris County, Texas

Gbade Ogungbade, DVM, PhD
Health Services and Health Policy and Management Sciences
Population Health Research Institute
Houston, Texas

John Balogun, MD, MPH
Disease Control and Preventive Health Services
University of Texas, School of Public Health
Houston, Texas

Joan Nwuli, JD
Health Policy and Management Sciences
Nwuli & Associates Law Firm
Houston, Texas

INTRODUCTION

Public health can be defined as what we as a society can do to remain healthy. This broad notion of public health is indicative of the shared responsibility of the governmental agencies, public and private sectors, and the community in meeting the demands of the core functions of public health, namely assessment, policy, and assurance. These core functions are fused into the essential public health services: (1) health services monitoring and identification of community health needs; (2) diagnoses and investigation of health problems and health hazards in the community; (3) informing, educating, and empowering people about health issues; (4) mobilizing community partnerships to identify and solve health problems; (5) enforcing laws and regulations that protect and ensure safety; (6) linking people with needed personal health services and ensuring the provision of health care when otherwise unavailable; (7) ensuring a competent public health and personal healthcare workforce; (8) evaluating effectiveness, accessibility, and quality of personal and population-based health services; and (9) researching new insights and innovative solutions to health problems.

The core functions of public health and the essential public health services serve as the reference point for the core disciplines and cross-cutting areas in public health. The competencies in these core areas are indicative of the broad knowledge of public health in fulfilling its substance as declared by the Institute of Medicine in *The Future of Public Health*: disease control prevention and health promotion. The core competencies simply set the path regarding the volume of knowledge, attitude, and skills required of graduates of public health in delivering public health direct services, research, and teaching.

There is a need to standardize these core disciplines in terms of the core competencies in order to administer an examination that will fairly test knowledge and performance in these core disciplines and their cross-cutting areas. Using the core disciplines in public health and the cross-cutting areas (professionalism, leadership, systems thinking, program planning, diversity and culture, and public health biology), we reviewed public health knowledge and practice with the intent to provide candidates with the information needed to obtain a high yield in the National Public Health Certification Examination.

The National Public Health Certification Examination is based on the core competencies (epidemiology, biostatistics, behavioral and social sciences, environmental sciences and health policy, and management sciences) and the cross-cutting areas (communication and informatics, diversity and culture, leadership, public health biology, professionalism, programs planning, and systems thinking). The examination, which is computer based, comprises 200 multiple-choice questions to be taken in 4.5 hours.

This book is not a substitute for the recommended textbooks used in these various public health disciplines. To benefit from this book, graduates of public health are expected to have had a good exposure to these core disciplines prior to graduation. If less time was dedicated to these areas, readers or candidates for the certification examination will find this book useful as well, but it may initially appear to be challenging. Therefore, for optimal success in using this review, we recommend that candidates read these materials at least twice prior to attempting the questions at the end of the chapters, and then re-read the chapters. Perhaps the most effective way to attempt the question in the last chapter (practice test) is to allow yourself 72 seconds to answer each question; as you proceed, indicate your answer beside each question. By complying with these suggestions, you will be approximating the time limits imposed by the Examination Board. After answering all the questions in the practice test, spend some time verifying your answers by carefully reading the explanations. Although you may pay much attention to the questions you answered incorrectly, you should read all explanations if provided or return to the sections within the text to verify the accuracy of the answer. However, if after reading the explanation and the illustrations in the text, you feel you need more information about the materials covered, you should consult the references indicated with the explanations or other sources of similar information judged to be accurate.

Finally, because public health is an ever-changing science, we have consulted with information judged to be reliable at the time of the presentation of these materials. In spite of this, and because of the possibility of human error, the author, contributors, and publisher cannot be held responsible for any errors resulting from the use of this information. Therefore, readers are advised to consult other texts for the confirmation of the data presented herein.

We sincerely welcome suggestions, criticisms, and remarks for improvement of this review as examination recall materials become available. Therefore, all suggestions should be addressed to: Team@popmedintegrate.org.

PUBLIC HEALTH CERTIFICATION EXAMINATION REVIEW PRETEST*

CPH SAMPLE QUESTIONS

Directions: There are 18 questions in this test, ALL of which must be attempted. The questions are either multiple choice or matching. Please select the best response. The time allowed is 20 minutes.

Questions 1–3 (Vignette)

A study investigated the effects of radiation exposure to fallout from the Hanford Nuclear site in Washington State in the 1940s and 1950s and subsequent development of thyroid cancer among persons exposed as children and adolescents. Scientists used birth data from the study area to trace and contact subjects to participate in the study. Screening consisted of thyroid palpation, ultrasonography of the thyroid gland, and measurement of hormone concentrations in serum and urine. Individual thyroid radiation doses were estimated from interview data covering place of residence and dietary histories. As a result of screening, 19 subjects were diagnosed with thyroid cancer.

1. Which of the following terms best describes the type of study design? E

- **a.** Case-control
- **b.** Cross-sectional
- **c.** Ecological
- **d.** Prospective cohort
- **e.** Retrospective cohort

*The 18 sample test questions are taken from the National Board of Public Health Examiners' Web site at www.publichealthexam.org. The annotations for the answers that follow are provided by the author.

2. Which of the following is the most appropriate measure of the effect of this type of study?

- **a.** Correlation coefficient
- **b.** Odds ratio
- **c.** Prevalence odds ratio
- **d.** Regression coefficient
- **e.** Risk ratio

3. Which of the following terms is most appropriate to describe the cases of thyroid cancer identified during the first screening in this study?

- **a.** Incident
- **b.** Interval
- **c.** Prevalent
- **d.** Recurrent
- **e.** Concurrent

Questions 4–6 (Vignette)

A pilot study is conducted to determine whether a new drug effectively decreases cholesterol levels over a six-week period. Twelve subjects are enrolled, and serum cholesterol levels are measured before and after the six-week treatment period. Investigators plan to use a paired *t*-test to determine whether the drug was effective in reducing cholesterol levels.

4. The paired *t*-test is more appropriate for analysis of the results than a two-sample *t*-test for which of the following reasons?

- **a.** Dependence between the pretest and posttest measurements
- **b.** Elimination of noise due to confounders
- **c.** Heterogeneous variances of the two groups
- **d.** Non-randomness of the timing of the measurements
- **e.** Potential non-normality of the response

5. Which of the following are the degrees of freedom in the paired *t*-test?

a. 9
b. 10
c. 11
d. 12
e. 13

6. If the *p* value was calculated to be 0.015, which of the following would be the most appropriate interpretation of the *p* value?

a. The probability of seeing a result as unusual as the observed under the alternate hypothesis is very small
b. The probability of seeing a result as unusual as the observed under the null hypothesis is very small
c. The probability that the alternate hypothesis is false is very small
d. The probability that the alternate hypothesis is true is very small
e. The probability that the null hypothesis is true is very large

Questions 7 and 8 (Vignette)

The ministry of health of a developing country is considering the nationwide implementation of a test using biomarkers to screen for breast cancer. The test is delivered to health clinics in two similar regions of the country with the following results:

	Region A	**Region B**
Specificity	70%	80%
Sensitivity	85%	95%

The positive and negative predictive values are different between the 2 regions.

7. Which of the following is the most likely cause of the difference in the test's sensitivity and specificity between the two regions?

- **a.** The incidence of the disease is different between the two regions
- **b.** Length-biased sampling has occurred
- **c.** The prevalence of disease is different between the two regions
- **d.** The test is detecting the disease earlier in its natural history in one of the regions
- **e.** The test was not administered in similar conditions in the two regions

8. Which of the following is the most likely cause of the differences in the test's predictive values between the two regions?

- **a.** The incidence of the disease is different between the two regions
- **b.** Length-biased sampling has occurred
- **c.** The prevalence of disease is different between the two regions
- **d.** The test is detecting the disease earlier in its natural history in one of the regions
- **e.** The test was not administered in similar conditions in the two regions

9. A community-based study of a program to increase physical activity is conducted, and the findings are evaluated. A small *p* value with an estimate is reported. Which of the following is the best interpretation of the result?

- **a.** It is likely the estimate differs from the true value because of bias
- **b.** It is likely the estimate differs randomly and systematically from the norm because of inter-rater variability
- **c.** It is unlikely the estimate differs from the average because of chance
- **d.** It is unlikely the estimate differs from the expected value because of confounding
- **e.** It is unlikely the estimate differs from the expected value because of random variability

10. Which of the following statements best describes an intent-to-treat analysis?

- **a.** Analysis compared characteristics of participants who did versus did not adhere to the randomized treatment
- **b.** Analysis excluded all participants who did not adhere to the assigned randomized treatment
- **c.** Analysis maintained the original randomized assignment of treatments in the definition of intervention and control groups
- **d.** Analysis reorganized participants into intervention and control groups based on their actual participation

11. A study is conducted to examine whether elderly women in at-home care settings maintain more cognitive ability than women who are residents of skilled nursing care facilities. Two groups of 30 elderly women are recruited independently. One group includes women living at home with a caregiver; the second group includes women living in skilled nursing care facilities. The women are asked to perform a task and then receive a score on the execution of the task (high scores indicate higher cognitive functioning). Which of the following is the most appropriate approach for analyzing the data?

- **a.** Chi square (χ^2) test
- **b.** Correlation analysis
- **c.** Paired *t*-test
- **d.** Trend test
- **e.** Two-sample *t*-test

12. A study is conducted to evaluate the relationship between pet ownership and having depressive symptoms. Seventy (70) participants are recruited. Each subject is identified as a current pet owner or non-pet owner. Participants are categorized as having or not having symptoms of depression. Which of the following is the most appropriate method to evaluate the association between pet ownership and having depressive symptoms in this population?

A

a. Chi square (χ^2) test
b. Correlation analysis
c. Paired *t*-test
d. Trend test
e. Two-sample *t*-test

13. The epidemic of methyl mercury poisoning in Minamata, Japan, in the 1950s illustrated contamination of which of the following?

a. Dairy product
b. Feed grain
c. Fish
d. Soil
e. Water

Questions 14–18 (Matching)

For each public health scenario, select the most appropriate lead organization (a–e).

a. Bill and Melinda Gates Foundation
b. Centers for Disease Control and Prevention
c. Local public health agencies
d. National Institutes of Health
e. State public health agencies

14. Focuses on crisis-oriented infectious diseases such as anthrax diagnosed in postal workers

15. Focuses on basic sciences research aimed at curing human diseases such as investigating the use of statin drugs to reduce the incidence of Alzheimer's disease

16. Primarily focuses on improving global health, addressing diseases such as HIV, malaria, and tuberculosis

17. Holds the primary constitutional authority to address policies concerning improvement of birth outcomes, including birth weight, preterm births, and infant mortality and morbidity

18. Focuses on day-to-day operations of public health clinics

ANNOTATED ANSWERS

1. The correct answer is **E** (retrospective cohort study design). Cohort studies are traditionally classified as (a) prospective and (b) retrospective, depending on the temporal relationship between the initiation of the study and the outcome (occurrence of disease or event of interest). A design is considered a retrospective cohort, which also is termed historical cohort or nonconcurrent prospective study, if the exposures and the outcomes of interest (disease, for example) have already occurred prior to the initiation of the study. In prospective design, the exposure, which defines the cohort, has occurred in the exposed group prior to the initiation of the study but the outcome (disease) has not occurred. In this context, both groups are followed to assess the incidence rate of the disease, comparing the exposed to the unexposed. Both designs compare the exposed group to the unexposed group to assess

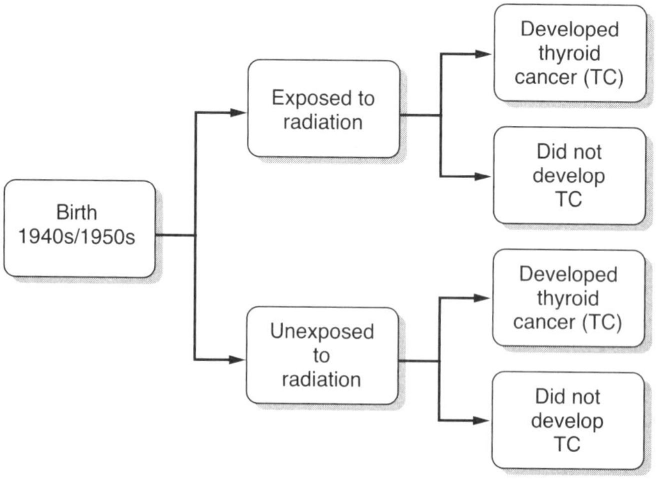

Figure 1 Illustration of retrospective cohort design. Thyroid cancer had occurred prior to the initiation of the study, and both the exposed and unexposed are screened for thyroid cancer and compared with respect to the risk of thyroid cancer in the exposed (radiation) versus the unexposed.

the measure of effect. However, the main distinction between these two designs is the calendar time. In the retrospective design, as illustrated in this vignette, exposure to radiation is ascertained from birth data (medical record) and the outcome (thyroid cancer) at the beginning of the study (no follow-up).

Cross-sectional studies also termed surveys and prevalence studies are designed to assess both the exposure and outcome simultaneously. However, since exposure and disease status are measured at the same point in time (snapshot), it is difficult, if not impossible, to distinguish whether the exposure preceded or followed the disease, and thus cause and effect relationships are not certain, lacking temporal sequence.

A case-control design classifies subjects on the basis of outcome (disease and non-disease or comparison group) and then looks backward to identify the exposure. This design could be prospective as well. In this design, the history or previous events for both cases and comparison groups are assessed in an attempt to identify the exposure or risk factors for the disease.

2. The correct answer is **E** (effect measure/size/point estimate in cohort design). Cohort studies are designed to determine whether there is an association between the exposure and the development of a disease. This association is determined by the ratio of the risk of disease in the exposed to the risk of disease in the unexposed. The relative risk (RR) is computed by risk in exposed/risk in unexposed. Relative risk can be computed as well by incidence in the exposed/incidence in unexposed. Further, risk ratio (RR) is often used, which is the disease risk in exposed/disease risk in the unexposed. In retrospective cohort design, risk ratio is an appropriate measure of effect.

3. The correct answer is **C** (prevalent cases and retrospective design). Incidence refers to new cases, whereas prevalence refers to existing cases (both old and new cases). In this example the screening test does not differentiate between old and new cases. The cases diagnosed with thyroid cancer constitute both old and new cases, and hence it is very appropriate to identify them as prevalent cases.

4. The correct answer is **E** (assumptions and rationale for paired *t*-test). The *t*-test is an appropriate statistical test that compares the means of two groups of observations. The observations should be randomly assigned to the two groups, so that any difference in response is due to the treatment and not to other factors. The paired *t*-test compares two paired groups so one can make inferences about the size of the average treatment effect, implying the average difference between the paired measurements. The rationale for using a paired *t*-test is to control for experimental variability as well as potential nonnormality of the response. Thus by analyzing only the differences, a paired *t*-test corrects for those sources of scatter or variability.

5. The correct answer is **C** (estimation of degrees of freedom in *t*-test). When the population standard deviation is unknown and the sample size is less than 30 ($n < 30$), the distribution of the test statistic cannot be guaranteed to be normal. Hence, the test statistic can be said to conform to a *t* distribution. The *t* distribution is similar to the standard normal distribution in that it is symmetrically distributed around a mean value. However, the *t* distribution varies from the standard normal, in that its standard deviation is determined by the number of degrees of freedom. Degrees of freedom (DF) are calculated from the size of the sample. Simply, DF is a measure of the amount of information from the sample data that has been utilized. Thus whenever a paired *t*-test statistic is calculated from a sample, one degree of freedom is used up. In this example, the DF $= n - 1 \rightarrow (12 - 1) = 11$.

6. The correct answer is **B** (*p* value interpretation). The level at which a result is considered significant is known as the type I error rate or α. A *p* value is a measure of how much evidence one has against the null hypothesis. The smaller the *p* value, the more evidence one has. One may combine the *p* value with the significance level to make a decision on a given test of hypothesis. A *p* value is not the probability that the null hypothesis is true but should be seen as the measure of the strength of the evidence provided by the data in favor of the null hypothesis.

Table 1 Hypothesis Testing and Relationship between Type I and Type II Errors

	Null hypothesis	
Test results	**False**	**True**
Significant	Power	Type I error
Non-significant	Type II error	

7. The correct answer is **E** (diagnostic test). Sensitivity and specificity are properties of a diagnostic test and should be consistent when the test is used in similar patients and in similar settings. Predictive values, though related to the sensitivity and specificity of the test, will vary with the prevalence of the condition or disease being tested. The difference in the sensitivity and specificity of the test is most likely a result of the test not being administered in similar conditions (patients and settings).

8. The correct answer is **C** (relationship between disease prevalence, sensitivity, specificity, and predictive values). The prevalence simply means the probability of the condition before performing the test (i.e., pretest probability). The predictive values refer to the probability of the disease being present or absent after obtaining the results of the test. Using the 2 × 2 table, positive predictive value (PPV) is the proportion of those with a positive test who have the disease ($a / (a + b)$) while the negative predictive value (NPV) is the proportion of those with a negative test who do not have the disease ($d / (c + d)$). The predictive values will vary with the prevalence of the disease or condition being tested for. Therefore the probability of the diseases before (prevalence) and the probability of disease after (predictive value) will be interrelated, with the differences in predictive values driven by the differences in the prevalence of the disease.

9. The correct answer is **E** (*p* value interpretation and sampling variability). The *p* value gives an indication of how plausible the null hypothesis is, but it is *not* the probability of the null hypothesis being true. Simply, the *p* value is the probability of observing a result as extreme as or more extreme than the one actually observed by chance alone; that is, if the null hypothesis is true.

Table 2 Hypothesis Testing and Type I Error

	Truth	
Test results	**No association**	**Association**
No association	Correct	Type II error
Association	Type I error*	Correct

* *p* value is the probability of a type I error.

10. The correct answer is **C** (analysis strategies in intervention trial—intent to treat versus efficacy analysis). Two types of analytic approaches are often used in clinical trials (randomized), namely efficacy and intent-to-treat. The latter is a method of analysis used in which all patients randomly assigned to one of the treatments arms are analyzed together, regardless of whether or not they completed or received that treatment. On the other hand, efficacy analysis is performed only on those who comply with the assigned treatment.

11. The correct answer is **E** (test statistic and hypothesis testing). The unpaired *t*-test, two sample *t*-test, or independent-samples *t*-test compares the means of two groups, assuming that data are sampled from Gaussian populations (normal distribution). If the *p* value is small (< 0.05), for instance, then it is unlikely that the observed difference is due to random variability or sampling error.

12. The correct answer is **A** (test statistic and hypothesis testing). The chi-square statistic is a non-parametric analytic method used to compare the observed frequency of some observation with an expected frequency. The comparison of observed and expected frequencies is used to calculate the value of the chi-square statistic, which in turn can be compared with the distribution of chi-square to make an inference about a statistical issue such as the relationship between pet ownership and depressive symptoms, hypertension and sodium intake, maternal preconception weight and low birth weight, etc.

Table 3 Choice of Statistical Test for Selected Data Types

Data Distribution	Groups (number)	Test statistic—independent sample	Test statistic—paired sample
Continuous (non-normal)	2	Mann–Whitney U test	Wilcoxon signed-rank test
Continuous (normal)	2 ($n > 30$)	*t*-test	Paired *t*-test

Table 3 Choice of Statistical Test for Selected Data Types *(cont.)*

Data Distribution	Groups (number)	Test statistic—independent sample	Test statistic—paired sample
Normal (non-normal)	≥ 3	Kruskal–Wallis test	Friedman test
Normal (normal)	≥ 3	ANOVA*	Repeated measures ANOVA
Ordinal	2	Mann–Whitney U test	Wilcoxon signed-rank test
	≥ 3	Kruskal–Wallis test	Friedman test
Nominal	2	Fisher exact test, Chi square	McNemar test
	≥ 3	Pearson chi-square test	Cochran Q test
Binary outcome	—	Unconditional logistic regression	Conditional logistic regression
Continuous	—	Linear regression	—

*Analysis of variance = ANOVA

13. The correct answer is **C** (environmental contaminants). In 1907 the Chisso Corporation built a factory in the small fishing village of Minamata, Japan, along the shore of Minamata Bay. The fish populations began to decline in 1925, and by 1950 fish began to float to the surface and shellfish and other aquatic organisms began to perish as well.

14–18. The correct answers are **B**, **D**, **A**, **E**, and **C**, respectively (agencies and public health responsibilities). The CDC focuses on crisis-oriented infectious diseases, such as anthrax diagnosed in postal workers. The NIH focuses on basic sciences research aimed at curing human diseases, such as investigating the use of statin drugs to reduce the incidence of Alzheimer's disease. The Bill and Melinda Gates Foundation primarily focuses on improving global health diseases, such as HIV, malaria, and tuberculosis. State health departments hold the primary constitutional authority to address policies concerning improvement of birth outcomes, including birth weight, preterm births, and infant mortality and morbidity. Local health departments (county and city) focus on day-to-day operations of public health clinics.

Chapter 1

Public Health Science: Principles and Practice

Larry Holmes, Jr., Doriel Ward, Jennifer Thompson, and John Balogun

OVERVIEW

Public health emerged from the need to provide clean and safe water and protect the population from contaminated food in an attempt to reduce morbidity and mortality from infectious diseases; it remains a collective attempt by the government, public and private sectors, and individual communities to ensure that we as a society or people stay healthy. Whereas there are many definitions of public health, simply, *public health* is the science and art of disease, disability and injury prevention, and health promotion at a population level.

This chapter reviews the mission, goal, substance, and core functions of public health. To achieve these core functions, the framework of public health integrates both the substance of public health, which are disease prevention and health promotions, and the essential public health services, namely, (a) health services monitoring and identification of community health needs; (b) diagnoses and investigation of health problems and health hazards in the community; (c) informing, educating, and empowering people about health issues; (d) mobilizing community partnerships to identify and solve health problems; (e) enforcing laws and regulations that protect and ensure safety; (f) linking people with needed personal health services and ensuring the provision of health care when otherwise unavailable; (g) ensuring a competent public health and personal health care workforce; (h) evaluating effectiveness, accessibility, and quality of personal and population-based health services; and (i) researching new insights and innovative solutions to health problems.

The history of public health is reviewed, with the main focus on the achievement of public health during the 21st century, namely, (a) motor vehicle safety, (b) safer workplaces, (c) infectious disease control, (d) decline in coronary artery disease and stroke mortality, (e) safer and healthier food, (f) healthier mothers and babies, (g) family planning, (h) fluorination of drinking water, (i) vaccination, and (j) recognition of tobacco as a health hazard. The challenges of public health today are also briefly mentioned: (a) aging U.S. population with the associated chronic diseases and disabilities, (b) climate changes and global warming, (c) bioterrorism and disaster preparedness, and (d) increasing health disparities.

I. Notion of Public Health

A. Public health is the interdisciplinary science and art of disease, disability, injury prevention, and control in the human population.
   1. Public health focuses on preventing diseases, prolonging life, and promoting physical and mental health, sanitation, personal hygiene, infection control, and organization of health services.
   2. Public health also focuses on enhancing health in human populations through organized community efforts.
   3. Public health is what we, as a society, do collectively to ensure that people can be healthy.

B. The *mission* of public health is to fulfill society's interest in ensuring conditions in which the people (community) can be healthy.

C. The *goal* of public health is to promote population health through shared responsibility, organized efforts, and managed care.

D. The *core functions* of public health agencies at all levels of government, are *assessment* of needs and health status, *policy* development, and *assurance* of public health services.

E. Public health *substance* is disease, injury, and disability control and prevention, and health promotion, achieved through organized community effort.

F. *Health* is defined by the World Health Organization (WHO) as the state of physical, mental, and social well-being, not the mere absence of a disease.

G. *Health care* is the prevention, treatment, and management of illness and the preservation of mental and physical well-being through the services offered by the medical, nursing, and allied health professions.

   1. According to the WHO, health care embraces all the goods and services designed to promote health, including "preventive, curative and palliative interventions, whether directed to individuals or to populations."

II. Public Health versus Medicine

A. *Public health* is concerned with the *community or population,* including animal populations (veterinary public health).

B. *Medicine* is concerned *with individual patients.*

C. *Public health* focuses on *preventing* illness, disabilities, and injuries.

D. *Medicine* focuses on the *treatment* of individual patients.

III. Public Health Approach to Disease and Disability and Injury Prevention

Table 1-1 The Stages in Public Health Initiative in Disease, Disabilities, and Injuries Prevention at the Population Level

Stages	Description
Health problem ascertainment	Clear and unambiguous definition of the health problem
Risk/protective factors identification	Postulated and researched risk factors
Intervention development	Intervention design and pilot
Intervention implementation	Intervention conduct
Program monitoring and evaluation	Data collection, analysis, and interpretation and results dissemination

IV. Core Functions of Public Health and Essential Public Health Services

A. Core Functions of Public Health

Table 1-2 The Core Functions of Public Health

Core Function	Description
Assessment	Systematic collection Assembling data (processing) Data analyses Dissemination of information on the health of the community, including health status statistics, community health needs, and epidemiologic and other studies of health problems
Policy development	The process by which society makes: ▪ Decisions about problems ▪ Chooses goals and the proper means to reach them ▪ Handles conflicting views about what should be done ▪ Allocates resources
Assurance	Provision of high-quality services, including personal health services, needed for the protection of public health are available and assessable to all persons ▪ Proper allocation of state, federal, and local resources for public health ▪ Availability of information on how to obtain and comply with health services requirements

B. Essential Public Health Services
   1. Monitoring and identifying of community health needs.
   2. Diagnosing and investigating of health problems and health hazards in the community.
   3. Informing, educating, and empowering people about health issues.
   4. Mobilizing community partnerships to identify and solve health problems.
   5. Enforcing laws and regulations that protect and ensure safety.
   6. Linking people with needed personal health services and ensuring the provision of health care when otherwise unavailable.
   7. Ensuring a competent public health and personal health care workforce.
   8. Evaluating effectiveness, accessibility, and quality of personal and population-based health services.
   9. Researching new insights and innovative solutions to health problems.

V. Origin of Public Health

A. Early History
   1. Diversion of human waste to protect public health (Roman times).
   2. Variolation (subcutaneous inoculation of attenuated pustule material in patients) following smallpox epidemic around 1000 B.C. (Chinese).
   3. Vaccination to treat smallpox by Edward Jenner (1820s).
   4. Removing dead bodies to prevent bacterial infection during the Black Death in Europe (14th century).
   5. Quarantine to mitigate infectious diseases (Medieval Europe).
   6. Development of the miasma theory of disease after cholera pandemic in Europe (1829–1851).

B. Modern History

1. Identification of polluted water well as the source of cholera epidemic in London in 1854 (John Snow). This indicated a transition from miasma theory of disease to the germ theory and was the foundation of the science of epidemiology.
2. Observation of microorganisms as the cause of most infectious diseases (Anton van Leeuwenhoek, 1680).
3. Germ theory—disease, single pathogen—defines a one-to-one relationship between a microorganism and the occurrence of disease (Robert Koch, mid- to late-1880s).
4. Artificial vaccine production and the theory that specific transmissible pathogens are responsible for disease (Louis Pasteur, mid-1800s).
5. Infant mortality lowering in the United States using preventive methods (feed, bathe, and dress babies)—Sara Josephine Baker, 21st century.
6. Increase in average life span in 21st-century United States due to public health achievements in vaccination programs and control of infectious diseases, motor vehicle and occupational safety, improved family planning, drinking water fluorination, and smoking cessation programs.
7. HIV/AIDS epidemic (1980s) and global response to HIV/AIDS epidemic.
8. Emerging infectious diseases such as sudden acute respiratory syndrome (SARS) in 2002.
9. Increase in obesity and type II diabetes (USA, 1990–2000s).
10. Population-level risk factors—health disparities, inequality, poverty, and education (1980s).
11. New public health challenge to address health inequalities by addressing social determinants of health, thus narrowing and eliminating health disparities in gender, education, race, and age.

12. Advocate policies that promote the health of the whole population in an equitable pattern (USA, 2000s).
13. Socioeconomic and social determinants of health being highly recognized (WHO, 2003).
14. Terrorism and bioterrorism preparedness (2000s).
15. Natural disaster preparedness (Katrina in United States and Tsunami in Asia, 2000s).

Table 1-3 The History of Public Health

Name	Accomplishment	Date
Romans	Diversion of human waste to protect public health	
Chinese	Variolation following smallpox	1000 B.C.
Edward Janner	Vaccination to treat smallpox	1880s
John Snow	Identification of polluted water source in cholera epidemic in London	1854
Jakob Henle, Robert Koch	Disease causation based on germ theory	1880s
South Carolina	First water protection regulation	1671
South Carolina	First Health Officer	1712
South Carolina	Identification of swamp drainage as essential in stopping malaria	1881
Lemuel Shattuck	Review of sanitation practices, enforcement of sanitation code, and the establishment of the Massachusetts local Board of Health	1850
South Carolina	Establishment of the State Board of Health	1898
Jonas Salk	Polio vaccine development reducing the number of U.S. cases from 58,000 in 1952 to 5,000 in 1957	1955

VI. Modern Functions and Accomplishments of Public Health

A. Health surveillance, monitoring, and analysis (epidemiology and biostatistics—assessment core function).

B. Disease outbreak investigation, epidemic and disease risk factors (epidemiology and biostatistics—assessment core function).

C. Establishing, designing, and managing health promotion and disease prevention programs (policy science, epidemiology, biostatistics, behavioral sciences—policy development and assessment core functions).

D. Enabling and empowering communities to promote health and reduce inequalities (policy and management science, health promotion and health promotion practices—policy and assurance core functions).

E. Ensuring compliance with regulations and laws to protect and promote health (management and policy science—assurance core function).

F. Creating and sustaining federal, state, local, and private sector partnership to improve health and reduce health disparities (policy and management science—policy and assurance core functions).

G. Developing and maintaining a well-educated and well-trained, multidisciplinary public health task force.

H. Providing comprehensive and current information in the training of able future leaders into the field of public health.

I. Ensuring the effective performance of Healthy People 2010 objectives in improving health, preventing diseases, and eliminating health disparities.

J. Encouraging research, development, evaluation, and innovation.

K. Increasing quality assurance in public health functions.

Table 1-4 21st-Century Public Health Achievement in the United States

- Vaccination
- Motor vehicle safety
- Safer workplaces
- Control of infectious diseases—infant mortality reduction
- Decline in coronary health disease and stroke deaths—reduction in cigarette smoking
- Safer and healthier food—FDA enforcement of related federal public health laws
- Healthier mothers and babies—improvement in maternal and child health services
- Family planning
- Fluorination of drinking water
- Recognition of tobacco as a hazard

Source: Centers for Disease Control and Prevention, http://www.cdc.gov/tobacco/mm4812.pdf

VII. Core Areas and Disciplines of Public Health

A. Basic Sciences of Public Health

Table 1-5 Basic Sciences of Public Health: Discipline and Basic Components/Features, Basic Sciences

Discipline	Characteristics/Features
Epidemiology: Science of disease, injuries and disabilities distribution, determinants and prevention in the human and related animal populations	Assessment of disease, disabilities, and injuries Disease distribution in human and related animal populations ▪ Persons/animals ▪ Place ▪ Time

Table 1-5 Basic Sciences of Public Health: Discipline and Basic Components/Features, Basic Sciences *(continued)*

Discipline	Characteristics/Features
	Measures of disease frequency Appropriate study designs to answer the research question(s) Measures disease risk (relative risk, odds ratio, prevalence odds ratio, risk ratio, hazards ratio) Determines disease causation (Hill & Doll's criteria, meta-analysis, factual inference) Determines study validity through critique and other measures Evidence-based risk and protective factors identification
Biostatistics: Science of inferences on random sample	Quantification of disease, disabilities and injuries Sampling techniques and appropriate sample (decision on how many will be in the study) ▪ Response rate and attrition ▪ Power estimation Probability of performance/diagnostic test ▪ Sensitivity, specificity, predictive value Design and analysis techniques for observational and clinical trial studies Hypotheses testing (parametric and nonparametric) Role of statistics in epidemiologic/public health research Inferential statistics and studies recommendation

B. Applied Sciences of Public Health

Table 1-6 Basic Sciences of Public Health: Discipline and Basic Components/Features, Applied Sciences

Discipline	Characteristics/Features
Behavioral and social sciences: Multidisciplinary science of human actions and reactions	Health theories, models, and beliefs Behavioral risk and protective factors in disease Social determinants of diseases and racial disparities in screening, diagnosis, treatment, and prognosis Behavioral interventions (community-based intervention trials, education intervention, behavior modeling, and motivation to change behavior) Health promotions and risk avoidance (HIV/AIDS, chronic diseases, obesity, cancer, infant mortality, prenatal care, etc.)
Environmental and occupational health: Science of environmental influence on health and effect of working environment on disease, disabilities, and injuries	Impact of environment on human health, occupational injury, diseases, and mortality Environmental factors in health promotion ▪ Routes and effects of exposure to environmental hazards ▪ Assessment of environmental risk ▪ Methods of environmental modification Major sources of environmental hazards ▪ Air pollution ▪ Water pollution ▪ Solid waste ▪ Contaminated food ▪ Environmental factors ▪ Weaponized pathogens

Table 1-6 Basic Sciences of Public Health: Discipline and Basic Components/Features, Applied Sciences *(continued)*

Discipline	Characteristics/Features
	Nutritional environment ▪ Effect of under-nutrition and over-nutrition ▪ Effect of excessive caloric intake and inadequate physical activities on health and disease outcomes
Management and policy science: Decision making on intervention goal and resources allocation	Policy development and public health Factors affecting public health Administration of public health Goals of public health

VIII. Challenges of Public Health

A. Global Warming

1. Climate warming and human health with the consequences being:
    a. Emerging hyperthermia.
    b. Emerging infections.
    c. Heat stroke, especially in individuals with cardiovascular system compromization or diseases and the elderly.
    d. Cutaneous malignancy.
    e. Increase in air and water pollution, resulting in infectious diseases.
    f. Asthma and pulmonary congestion.
    g. These conditions are likely to involve the socioeconomically marginalized segments of the U.S. population, mainly ethnic/racial minorities.

B. Aging America
   1. Aging population predisposes to chronic disabilities and chronic disease and malignancies.
   2. Public health is charged with implementing programs to address lifestyle variables and decrease chronic disabilities and illnesses and promote successful aging and disease-free longevity.

C. Obesity and Overweight
   1. More than 66% of the U.S. population is overweight and obese; the consequences of obesity and overweight are:
      a. Type II diabetes.
      b. Cardiovascular diseases.
      c. Some cancers.
      d. Preterm and low birth weights, congenital anomalies, and infant mortality.
      e. Maternal morbidity (gestational diabetes, pre-eclampsia).
   2. Public health is charged with preventing obesity by behavioral intervention to address excessive caloric intake and enhance regular and moderate exercise.

D. Terrorism
   1. Whereas public health is not designed to control or prevent terrorism, public health is charged with the responsibility of responding to such attacks by coordinating services needed to reduce causalities and respond to the attack, thus preventing further damages to human health and loss of human lives.

E. Disaster Preparedness
   1. Disasters, which public health cannot control, and the response to the aftermath of such disasters remain the responsibilities of public health.
   2. A prompt response to disasters such as Katrina in New Orleans and tsunami in Asia requires a well-coordinated disaster preparedness effort from the public health services.

F. Health Disparities Elimination
   1. Healthy People 2010 focuses on health disparities elimination.
   2. Public health is charged with the responsibility of providing equitable preventive services to all sectors of the population, especially the socioeconomically marginalized, children, women, elderly, and racial and ethnic minorities.
   3. Realistically, the future of the U.S. population's health depends on the collective and shared effort of public health agencies to develop and enforce policies that will ensure the provision of health services to all at a population level, regardless of the ability to afford such services (e.g., immunization as primary prevention of vaccine-preventable diseases).

REVIEW QUESTIONS (MULTIPLE CHOICE)

Directions: Each of the following questions contains multiple suggested responses. Select the *one best* response to each question.

1. Which of the following statements is *incorrect* regarding public health?

- **a.** The focus of a public health intervention is to prevent rather than treat a disease through surveillance of cases and the promotion of healthy behaviors.
- **b.** Public health is fulfilling society's interest in ensuring conditions in which people can be healthy.
- **c.** Immunization programs and distribution of condoms are examples of public health measures to control disease at the population level.
- **d.** Public health is concerned with medical care rather than preventive services.
- **e.** Public health focuses on prevention research rather than biomedical research.

2. Which of the following statements is *inaccurate* regarding the history of public health?

- **a.** The miasmatic theory of diseases held that diseases such as cholera or the Black Death was caused by "bad air."
- **b.** Robert Koch postulated the germ theory of disease.
- **c.** John Snow, following the cholera epidemic in Central London in 1854, disproved the miasmatic theory of disease causation.
- **d.** Edward Jenner utilized vaccination in the 1880s to treat smallpox.
- **e.** Jonas Salk developed the Hepatitis B vaccine to prevent viral hepatitis infection in the United States in 1955.

3. A 45-year-old Hispanic-American women residing in San Antonio, Texas, has a history of breast cancer in her family. On a visit to her primary care physician, she is scheduled to undergo both breast and cervical cancer screening. These services are considered to be:

- **a.** Primary prevention
- **b.** Secondary prevention
- **c.** Tertiary prevention
- **d.** Routine medical examination
- **e.** None of the above

4. The Boston City Health Department plans to reduce exposure to cigarettes in order to decrease the incidence of bladder cancer among its residents by implementing tobacco education sessions at all schools in the city. This approach best describes:

- **a.** Health promotion
- **b.** Disease prevention
- **c.** Disease screening
- **d.** All of the above
- **e.** None of the above

5. The Centers for Disease Control and Prevention (CDC) assessed the rate of dental cavities among inner-city African-American children in Baltimore, Maryland, and recommended water fluorination. This approach is best described as:

a. Health promotion
b. Disease prevention
c. Disease screening
d. a and c only
e. None of the above

6. The San Francisco City Health Department decides to immunize all high school students against Hepatitis B. This decision denotes an action, logically taken, to prevent the development of Hepatitis B infection in this group of school children who are healthy and do not currently have a Hepatitis B viral infection. This approach to disease prevention constitutes an example of:

a. Tertiary prevention
b. Disease screening
c. Secondary prevention
d. Primary prevention
e. Disease prognosis
f. None of the above

7. Assessment and policy development in public health require an understanding of the causes of health problems at the population level and depends on the knowledge provided by biomedical sciences, social and behavioral sciences, and environmental sciences. Which of the following sciences of public health is/are the basis for the assessment function of public health?

a. Management and policy science
b. Epidemiology
c. Public health biology
d. Biostatistics
e. b and d only
f. None of the above

8. Public health focus is on preventive measures, which makes its goal more abstract than medicine, rendering its achievement more difficult to recognize. As a public health professional, which of the following statements could most appropriately define your function?

a. Disease prevention and control
b. Disease identification
c. Health promotions
d. All of the above
e. None of the above

9. The graduate students at the Tulane University School of Public Health and Tropical Medicine are required by the Louisiana State Department of Health to determine the rate of prostate cancer among African-American males in the state. Which of the following are needed to achieve this public health core function of assessment?

a. Data collection
b. Data analysis and interpretation
c. Communication of information for action or intervention
d. a and b only
e. All of the above

10. The U.S. Department of Health and Human Services, through the Centers for Disease Control and Prevention, has proposed the role of public health in disaster preparedness such as Hurricane Katrina. Which of these is *not* the direct function of public health in disaster preparedness?

a. Prevention of disaster
b. Coordinating the response to disaster
c. Reducing the rate of causality through careful and strategic planning to treat the affected persons
d. Minimizing further casualties
e. None of the above

11. Global warming or climate change reflects the modern challenge to public health initiative in preventing diseases and promoting the health of the population. There are logical and practical health concerns as the consequence of global warming. Which of the following condition/s would you consider as the effect of such a climate change?

a. Emerging hyperthermia and heat stroke
b. Increase in cardiovascular diseases especially among the vulnerable populations
c. Increase in pulmonary disorders such as asthma
d. All of the above
e. None of the above

12. The Healthy People 2010 objectives call on public health to reduce health disparities. As a public health professional entrusted with the responsibility of reducing health disparities in breast cancer, which of the following areas of disparities will be an important focus to you in arriving at this goal?

a. Education
b. Race/ethnicity
c. Income
d. Age
e. All of the above

13. Public health achievements are often unrecognized. If you are appointed the director of a state health department and are requested to convince the elected officials of the achievements of public health during the 21st century in this nation, which of the following would you consider as part of the *top 10* accomplishments of public health?

a. Routine use of vaccination and healthier mothers and babies
b. Improvement in motor vehicle safety and fluoridation of water
c. Safer workplaces and safer and healthier foods
d. Control of infectious disease and decline in deaths from heart disease and stroke
e. b and c only
f. All of the above

14. As a newly assigned director of a county health department, you are required to brief the commissioner's court on the challenges of public health in your county in order to prepare a long-term budget to address these issues. Given the general knowledge of what public health will be facing in the future, which of the following areas would you include in your briefing?

a. Emerging infectious disease such as AIDS/TB, antibiotics resistance, and foodborne pathogens
b. Aging and the related chronic disabilities and chronic diseases
c. Obesity and overweight and its consequences
d. Disaster and bioterrorism preparedness
e. b and c only
f. All of the above

15. You are recently appointed to direct the chronic disease prevention program for the elderly in the state of Illinois, and your goal at interview was morbidity compression. Which of the following interventions would you consider beneficial in your program?

a. Smoking cessation
b. Dietary modification
c. Physical activities
d. Recreational activities
e. a and c only
f. All of the above

ANNOTATED ANSWERS

1. The correct answer is **D** (mission and goal of public health). Public health definition remains complex. Broadly, the Committee for the Study of the Future of Public Health defines the mission of public health as fulfilling society's interest in assuring conditions in which people can be healthy. Public health is concerned with disease control and prevention at the population level and focuses on preventive research. Also, public health focuses on preventive services rather than medical care services (Institute of Medicine, *The Future of Public Health*, 1988, pp. 1–17).

2. The correct answer is **E** (history of public health). The history of public health reflects the notion of disease causation and the measures to prevent diseases at the population level. The miasmatic theory dominated public health for a long period and was disproved by the germ theory. Koch's postulate in the 1880s represented a great notion of disease causation for the germ theory. John Snow, respected as the father of epidemiology, attributed the cholera epidemic in London in 1854 to polluted water. Jonas Salk in 1955 discovered the polio vaccine, which resulted in a remarkable reduction of polio cases in the United States (Institute of Medicine, *The Future of Public Health*, 1988, pp. 56–71).

3. The correct answer is **B** (methods of prevention). Preventing the occurrence of an illness, disabilities, or injuries in the first place, by avoiding risk or predisposing factors, refers to primary prevention. This denotes an action such as immunization taken to prevent the development of a vaccine-preventable disease in a person without the disease in question. The objective of secondary prevention is to minimize the severity of illness or damage to an injury-causing event once the event has occurred. Also, secondary prevention is aimed at early detection of a disease, either through screening or case finding, followed by treatment or intervention (e.g., the routine testing of stool for occult blood to detect treatable colon cancer in the early stage of the natural history of the disease). Tertiary prevention is aimed at medical treatment and rehabilitation, as with a stroke, with the intent to restore, improve, and prevent further neurologic damage to the individual. Disease screening involves the identification of a subgroup of people who are at risk for having asymptomatic disease or who have a risk factor that predispose them to developing a disease or becoming injured (Gordis, L., *Epidemiology*, 3rd ed., 2004, pp. 5–6).

4. The correct answer is **A** (behavioral intervention and health promotion). Health promotion is an intervention that seeks to eliminate or minimize risk exposure by modifying behavior, thus improving and protecting health.

5. The correct answer is **B** (intervention and disease control). Disease prevention is any intervention, such as immunization, water chlorination, and fluorination, that is aimed at reducing or minimizing diagnosable conditions.

6. The correct answer is **D** (methods of prevention). *Primary prevention* denotes an action taken to prevent the development of a disease in a person who is well and does not have the disease in question. *Disease screening* is an action to identify those who are diseased, given the manifestation, and those who are not, given the absence of the manifestation. *Secondary prevention* denotes the identification of persons who have already developed early-stage Hepatitis B, for instance, through screening and early intervention. Identification of cases at an early stage in the natural history of the disease is indicative of the effectiveness of the intervention. *Disease prognosis* refers to the outcome of treatment following the diagnosis of the disease. *Tertiary prevention* involves treatment after disease (e.g., stroke) has been diagnosed and rehabilitation to prevent further health consequences (Schneider, M., *Introduction to Public Health*, 2nd ed., 2006, p. 12).

7. The correct answer is **E** (basic sciences of public health). *Epidemiology* and *biostatistics* or *biometry* are the basis of the assessment function of public health. Whereas epidemiology is involved in the design of study to assess the risk variable or determinants, statistics is essential in testing the hypothesis for possible inference, and statistical analysis is an integral part of an epidemiologic design. *Management and policy science* provide the basis for service provision and the evaluation of the public health programs, as well as the assurance that services are being provided and utilized by the population. *Public health biology* provides the information for the understanding of the disease or disabilities under assessment (Schneider, M., *Introduction to Public Health*, 2nd ed., 2006, pp. 8–9; U.S. Institute of Medicine, *The Future of Public Health*, 1988, p. 88).

8. The correct answer is **D** (core functions of public health). The Institute of Medicine describes the substance of public health as that of disease prevention and health promotion. The assessment function of public health denotes disease identification at the population level. All these represent the functions that are carried out by public health professionals, in attempting to quantify disease, injury, or disabilities at the population level (Institute of Medicine, *Healthy Communities*, 1996, p. 8).

9. The correct answer is **E** (core functions of public health). The assessment function of public health calls for epidemiologic surveillance, which involves continuous data collection, analysis, interpretation, and information dissemination prior to intervention (Institute of Medicine, *The Future of Public Health*, 1988, pp. 1–17).

10. The correct answer is **A** (the future and challenges of public health). Public health is challenged with increasing natural disasters, which are obvious threats to population health. The aftermath of hurricanes such as Katrina very clearly illustrate the deficiencies in the public health response to natural disaster. To prevent disaster is not a direct function of public health. Public health is charged with coordinating an effective response in minimizing further causalities, improving the health of the survivors, and preventing further casualties through the collective and shared responsibilities of governmental and private sectors (Schneider, M., *Introduction to Public Health*, 2nd ed., 2006, pp. 535–550).

11. The correct answer is **D** (public health and global warming). There is an association between seasonal variation and human health, including mental health. Extreme temperatures can result in failure in the thermoregulatory center, the hypothalamus, leading to death. Hospital data on admission and mortality indicate an increasing rate of deaths during extremely hot days, especially among the elderly, young children, and those with chronic diseases. Also, extreme temperature can lead to increases in air and water pollution and the subsequent infectious diseases such as West Nile virus, cholera, and Lyme disease (pathogens affiliated with high heat, as seen in summer). The physical effect of climate change is an alteration in the air temperature, thus increasing the concentration of ozone at ground level. Exposure to ozone, especially by those with already compromised cardiorespiratory function, may result in chest pain and pulmonary congestion (U.S. Global Change Research Program, A report of the National Assessment Synthesis Team, *Climate Change Impacts on the United States—The Potential Consequences of Climate Variability and Change*, http://www.usgcrp.gov/usgcrp/naac, accessed 11/12/2007).

12. The correct answer is **E** (health disparities and challenges of public health). The burden of disease is disproportionately shared in the United Sates as well as in other nations, including the United Kingdom. In the United Kingdom, where social class is obvious, the laborers are disproportionately affected compared with professional classes such as physicians, lawyers, etc. In the United States, where social class remains an unpopular notion in research settings, socioeconomic variance is used to describe health disparities, with the economically marginalized, which implies the ethnic minorities (mainly African Americans), associated with the greatest burden of disease. Health disparity is also affected by education, age, and gender. In the United States, the observed racial/ethnic disparities in health are realistically driven by socioeconomic variance (Centers for Disease Control and Prevention, *Eliminating Racial & Ethnic Health Disparities*, http://www.cdc.gov/omhd, accessed 11/15/2007).

13. The correct answer is **F** (public health accomplishments). The CDC noted the top 10 accomplishments of public health during the 20th century as (a) routine use of vaccination, (b) healthier mothers and babies, (c) improvement in motor vehicle safety, (d) fluoridation of water, (e) safer workplaces, (f) safer and healthier foods, (g) control of infectious disease, (h) decline in deaths from heart disease and stroke, (i) access to family planning and contraceptive services, and (j) recognition of tobacco use as a health hazard. Remarkably, the increase in life expectancy has been associated with these achievements, mainly, the decline in deaths due to heart disease and stroke as a result of tobacco education and lifestyle modification in this direction (Centers for Disease Control and Prevention, *MMWR*, 1999a, 48:241–243).

14. The correct answer is **F** (challenges of public health). Public health is threatened with the emerging infections and the antibiotic resistance associated with the changes in the enveloping proteins of these pathogens as they continue to mutate. The epidemic of obesity and overweight presents a great challenge to public health and requires research and behavioral interventions in addressing its behavioral and lifestyle components. Realistically, the life expectancy gained by this nation in the areas of heart disease and stroke as a result of tobacco cessation and lifestyle modification in this direction will be lost to the obesity epidemic. Public health agencies need to act now to reduce the epidemic of obesity and overweight. Aging is not a pathologic process but is associated with decline in the biologic system. To address successful aging, public health needs to prevent chronic diseases and chronic disabilities in the first place and compress morbidity. Therefore, achieving successful aging or disease-free longevity is a challenge to public health in any society with an increasingly aging population. The increasing disparities in health, with the racial/ethnic minorities (mainly African Americans) being disproportionately burdened, is indicative of the need to provide equitable public health services to such vulnerable populations. Public health is challenged with confronting health with politics and allocating resources to those who cannot afford health in our society (Riscia, P.M., *Prevention of*

Overweight and Obesity: Focus on Children and Adolescents; Ory, M.G., *Emerging Issues in Geriatric Care: Aging and Public Health Perspectives*; Glik, D.C., *Bioterrorism Preparedness: Workforce, Organizational, Resources, and Risk Communication Issues*—all presented at the American Public Health Association 132nd Annual Meeting, November 6–10, 2004, Washington, DC).

15. The correct answer is **F** (chronic disease and challenges of public health). Morbidity compression refers to the delaying of illness (chronic diseases and disabilities) into oldest old age, with instant mortality at age 90–100 years. Whereas aging is not a pathologic process, it is associated with decline in biologic functions, which could be delayed or improved by adequate lifestyle and health surveillance such as routine screening. An effective chronic disease program will benefit substantially from a well-designed intervention addressing cigarette and excessive alcohol consumption, dietary modification with emphasis on a low-fat diet and an increase in vegetable and fruit consumption, as well as 30–60 minutes of moderate exercise daily, because what matters for the aging biologic system is not the intensity of the exercise but the frequency, in the reconditioning of the cardiocirculatory system and the musculature (Ory, M.G., *Emerging Issues in Geriatric Care: Aging and Public Health Perspectives*, American Public Health Association 132nd Annual Meeting, November 6–10, 2004, Washington, DC).

Chapter 2

Principles and Methods of Epidemiology

Larry Holmes, Jr.

OVERVIEW

Epidemiology is simply a population-oriented discipline that quantifies and determines causes of health-related states or events, and applies this knowledge to prevention and control of health-related events in specified populations. Epidemiology had been traditionally defined as the study of the distribution and determinants of health-related events in the human population and the application of this knowledge to disease, disability, and injury control and prevention. As a basic science of public health, epidemiology is involved in the assessment and monitoring of health status at the population level and the application of these results in disease prevention and control. Specifically, epidemiology deals with (a) measurement of disease occurrence and frequency in the population; (b) identification of when, where, and within which population subgroups health-related events are more or less likely to occur; (c) determining the causes at the population level; (d) determining the mechanisms of causation, natural history, and the clinical course of the health-related events; and (e) application of the results to the prevention and control of disease and health-related events.

This chapter reviews the definition and role of epidemiology in public health in relation to the core functions of public health mainly, descriptive epidemiology which refers to, (a) place, (b) person, and (c) time. Measures of disease frequency and occurrence and types of epidemiologic designs are also discussed, (a) ecologic, (b) cross-sectional, (c) case-control, (d) cohort, and (e) experimental (clinical trial). Each epidemiologic design is followed by an in-depth review of the study description, measures of association or point estimate, and advantages and limitations of each design. Further, both internal and external validity of epidemiologic studies are reviewed, with emphasis on confounding, bias as systematic error, random error, effect measure modifier or interaction, and epidemiologic causal inference.

I. Definition of Epidemiology

A. Basic science of human public health that deals with the *distribution*, *determinants*, and *prevention* of disease, disabilities, and injuries in human populations.

1. Because public health is incomplete without animal health, the definition of epidemiology transcends human population and embraces animal populations, which is the focus of veterinary public health.

B. Study of the distribution and determinants of health-related states or events in *specified populations*, and the *application* of this study to the control of health problems.

1. *Distribution* implies the frequency (number, percentage, prevalence, rates, ratio, risk) and pattern (time, place, person) of health events in a population.
2. *Determinants* imply the causes, variables, and factors influencing the health-related events with respect to their occurrences.
3. *Specified population* implies the collective health of the population/people in a community setting in contrast to clinical medicine, which is concerned with the health of an individual patient.
4. *Application*: Whereas the primary role of epidemiology is not to control or prevent health-related events, it provides data for public health action in controlling and preventing diseases, disabilities, and injuries.

C. Epidemiology, which originates from *epidemic*, comes from the Greek word *epi* (upon) and *demos* (people). An epidemic implies the occurrence of disease, disability, and injury beyond the usual or the expected (out of proportion).

1. *Vignette*: A city of Notown, Texas, with a population of 246,000, normally has an incidence of Shigellosis of 5.0/1,000 during the summer months. In summer 2006, the incidence was 125.0/1,000. Is this an epidemic?
2. *Solution*: The occurrence of new cases (incidence) in 2006 clearly illustrates an epidemic of Shigellosis in Notown, Texas.

Table 2-1 Descriptive and Analytic Epidemiology

Descriptive Epidemiology	Analytic Epidemiology
Disease occurrence data with respect to time, place, and person	Disease causes data with respect to the rate of occurrence, the differences in rates, and why the differences occurred
Provides information on what, who, when, and where	Provides information on why and how

II. Role of Epidemiology in Public Health

A. Epidemiology focuses on the assessment of disease, disabilities, and injuries at the population level.

B. The knowledge gained from epidemiology is used to design intervention in order to prevent and control diseases, disabilities, and injuries at the population level.

C. Epidemiology is the tool for public health to use in its mission of disease control and health promotion. Epidemiology in public health is, therefore, a basic science providing analytic input to the understanding of health and health-related issues.

D. The focus of public health is to control and prevent disease, as well as promote health, whereas that of epidemiology is to assess the health condition involving the assessment of diseases, disabilities, and injuries, as well as health-related states.
   1. *Vignette*: The Delaware State Department of Health and Social Services is responding to increasing cases of childhood leukemia and lymphoma (hematological tumors). The chief epidemiologist proposes to examine the determinants of these tumors. The epidemiologist's role in this context is that of disease assessment, not control and prevention or health promotion. If the director of the department proposes to address the determinants of these hematological tumors by starting an intervention to eliminate environmental carcinogens, this approach illustrates the disease and health promotion role of public health.

Table 2-2 The Focus of Epidemiology and Public Health*

Epidemiology (Core Focus)	Public Health (Core Focus)
Assessment of diseases, disabilities, and injuries (health phenomena)	Control and prevention of diseases, disabilities, and injuries, as well as health promotion
Distribution (frequency) and determinants (risk and protective factors)	Intervention, design, and implementation to address disease, disabilities, and injuries, risk, and protective factors

* The primary focus of epidemiology is not to control and prevent diseases, disabilities, and promote population health. This is the primary function/role of public health.

III. History and Modern Concept of Epidemiology

Table 2-3 History of Modern Epidemiology

Person	Contribution to Disease Causation	Time (Period)
Hippocrates	Environmental and host factors in the development of a disease	Circa 400 B.C.
John Graunt—first epidemiologist, statistician, and demographer	Quantification of patterns of birth, death, and disease occurrence; bills of fertility, morbidity, and mortality on weekly count of death in London	1662
James Lind—surgeon with interest in epidemiology	Conducted one of the earliest experimental investigation on the treatment of scurvy; attributed causes of scurvy to moist air and diet	1747
William Farr—trained physician and self-taught mathematician	Described the state of health of the population, determinants of public health, as well as the application of the knowledge gained to the prevention and control of the disease	Mid-1800s
John Snow—physician	Established the cause and mode of communication of cholera in London	1854
British Medical Research Council	Streptomycin tuberculous trial	1940s
Bradford Hill and Richard Doll	Smoking as a causative agent in lung cancer	1950
Framingham Study	Foundation stone for cardiovascular risk factors (high blood pressure, elevated serum cholesterol level, physical activities, etc.)	1947–Present
Modern epidemiology	Health determinants at molecular and genetic levels; health determinants at biological and societal levels; penetration of the epidemiologic black box	21st century

IV. Models of Disease Causation

A. Causation refers to the process of an event (disease, disability, or injury) occurring as a result of either intrinsic or extrinsic factors acting individually or collectively.

B. Causal action of exposure comes before the subsequent development of disease as a consequence of exposure. Basis of longitudinal study where exposure data or information refers to an earlier time than that of disease, disability, or injury occurrence.

C. Intrinsic factor in disease causation simply refers to the host factor (organism). Example of this factor includes the immune system as well as the personality, social class membership, and race.

D. The extrinsic factor refers to the environmental factors, which are identified as biologic, social, and physical environments.

Table 2-4 Models of Disease Causation

Model	Description
Ecologic model	Disease occurs as a result of interrelationship between biological, social, and physical factors.
Epidemiologic triangle model*	Disease is caused by an imbalance between the host (intrinsic factor), agent, and environment.
Web of causation model	Diseases do not occur as a result of a single isolated factor but as a result of multiple factors interacting to predispose to disease (e.g., coronary artery disease, which is associated with diet, smoking, physical inactivity, estrogen replacement therapy, stress).

Table 2-4 Models of Disease Causation *(continued)*

Model	Description
Wheel model (man/environment interaction)	This model stresses the genetic makeup as the most prominent determinant of a disease.
	Ignores agent in the causation of the disease and places gene at the core of disease causation as well as incorporates social, biologic, and physical environment in the interpretation of disease process.
Causal pie (multi-causality)	Disease occurrence requires the joint action of component causes as "sufficient cause"; multitude of component causes.

* One of the most frequently used models, which claims that to understand the disease process, the environmental, the host, and the agent factors must be understood.

V. Measures of Disease Frequency

A. The measures of disease frequency include *ratios*, *proportion*, and *rates*.

B. Rates as used in public health involve incident rates, mortality rates, attack rates, and fatality rates.

   1. The basic measures of disease frequency in epidemiology are incidence and prevalence.

C. *Ratio* is one number (X) divided by another (Y). For example, the sex of adults attending a blood pressure screening clinic could be compared in this way (e.g., male/female; male/male + female).

D. *Proportion*: It is a type of ratio, but the numerator is included in the denominator.

   1. The distinction between a ratio and proportion, therefore, implies that the proportion represents the relationship between X and Y.

E. *Rate* is a type of proportion and is a measure of occurrence of events in a population over time.
   1. Time is therefore an integral part of the denominator in rate.
   2. Rate = Number of cases or events occurring during a given time period/Population at risk during the same time period $\times 10^n$.

F. *Vignette*: During the first 12 months of Nostate surveillance for AIDS malignancy (AM), the Health Department received 2,166 case reports that specified sex; 1,000 cases were in females, 1,166 in males. How will you calculate the female-to-male ratio for AM? In addition, how will you calculate the proportion of males with AM?
   1. *Ratio computation*: (1) Identify the number of AM cases of females (X) and the number of AM cases of males (Y). (2) Compute the ratio by using the basic formula: X (cases in females)/Y (cases in males). (3) Substituting for X and Y → 1,000/1,166 = 0.86:1.
      a. Therefore, there was less than 1 female patient for each male patient who reported for AM to the Health Department.
   2. *Proportion computation*: (1) Identify the number of AM cases of females (X), and the number of AM cases of females and males (Y). (2) Compute the proportion by using the basic formula: X (cases in females)/Y (cases in females and males). (3) Substituting for X and Y → 1,000/2,166 = 0.46.
      a. Therefore, less than 5 out of every 10 AM cases were in females.

G. Ratios and proportions are used to characterize populations by age, sex, race, exposure, etc.

H. Rates, ratios, and proportions are used to describe morbidity, mortality, and natality health and human conditions.

VI. Measures of Disease Occurrence

A. Comparing disease frequency involves measuring disease occurrence.

B. Measures of disease occurrence most frequently used in epidemiology are *risk*, *incidence rates*, and *prevalence*.

C. *Risk* refers to the probability that an individual or group of persons will develop a given disease.
   1. If the total number of persons in a population (Notown) equals *T*, and *D* represents the number of people out of the *T* population who develop the disease (AIDS malignancy [AM]) during the period of time, the proportion *D/T* represents the average risk of developing AM in the population during that period.

D. The *basic formula for risk* computation is: *D/T* = Number of subjects developing the disease or the event of interest during a time period/Number of subjects followed for that time period.

E. The *average risk* of a disease in a population is interchangeable with the *incidence proportion* as well as the *cumulative incidence* (CI) of the disease.
   1. CI is the proportion of the population that becomes diseased or presents with the event of interest over a specified period of time.
   2. Average risk of getting a disease over a period of time, which is the probability of getting a disease.
   3. Adequate measure when there are small or no losses to follow-up.
   4. The basic formula for CI is: Number of new cases of disease or event of interest or related health factor/Number in the population of interest, over a specific time period.

F. *Incidence rate* (IR) or incidence density (ID) is a measure of disease frequency or simply risk. Unlike cumulative incidence or average risk which ignores the concept of competing risk, thus underestimating the point estimate, the denominator of IR consists of the sum of the different times that each individual was at risk.

G. Rates can be used to estimate risk only when the period of follow-up is short and the rate of the disease over that interval is relatively constant.
   1. IR takes into account the competing risk by modeling the disease occurrence with the Person-Time (P-T) of observation.

H. IR or *incidence density* (ID) is the occurrence of new cases of disease or events of interest that arise during P-T of observation.
   1. The basic formula for IR is Number of subjects developing the disease or events of interest (new cases)/Total time experienced by the subjects followed (P-T) of observation.
   2. *Vignette*: Consider that in Newcity, 35,000 women were at risk for postmenopausal breast cancer and contributed 250,000 person-years of follow-up. If there were 1,500 incident cases during the 10-year follow-up, what would be the incidence density for breast cancer in this population?
   3. *Computation*: (1) Identify the number of cases during the time period (*A*) and identify the total person-time of observation (follow-up) (*B*). (2) Apply the basic formula, *A/B*. (3) Substituting → 1,500/ 250,000 = 600.0 per 100,000 per year.
   4. *Cumulative incidence* is related to *incidence rate* by the formula CI = IR × *T*, where *T* is the specified period of time.
   5. Risk is related to IR and is mathematically given by Risk = IR × *T*.

I. *Prevalence proportion* (P) measures the frequency of the existing disease (disease status).
   1. Two types of prevalence measures are common in epidemiology:
      a. *Point prevalence* (proportion of the population that is diseased (new cases, current cases, old cases) at a single point in time.
      b. *Period prevalence* (proportion of the population that is diseased during a specified duration of time), for example, during the year 2006.

J. The denominator for the point prevalence is the estimated population at the point in time, whereas the denominator of the period prevalence is the estimated population at mid-interval.

K. *Prevalence* is influenced by *time*.
   1. The longer the duration of the disease, the greater the prevalence.

2. Prevalence is influenced by both incidence rate and disease duration.
3. The relationship between prevalence and incidence rate is given by P = IR × *D*, where *D* is the duration of the disease or the event of interest (applicable to low disease prevalence, i.e., less than 10%).

L. When the prevalence of the disease is not low, the relationship between the prevalence and incidence rate is given by P = ID (1 + ID), where *I* = incidence and *D* = the duration of the disease.

1. The basic formula for *point prevalence* is Number of existing cases of disease or event of interest/Number in total population, at the point in time.
2. *Period prevalence* is given by the formula Number of existing cases of disease or event of interest/Number in total population (estimated population at mid-interval).

VII. Uses of Incidence and Prevalence Data

Table 2-5 Uses of Incidence and Prevalence Data in Public Health

Prevalence

Important and useful in the planning and monitoring of public health services (facilities, personnel, manpower)

Expresses the burden of health-related events in a specified population

Useful in determining the extent of the health-related events

Substitution for the calculation of the impact of the health-related events in the absence of incidence data

- Not a good estimator of incidence

Point prevalence is useful in tracking changes of health-related events in a population over time

Table 2-5 Uses of Incidence and Prevalence Data in Public Health *(continued)*

Incidence
Important in estimating disease etiology
Provides direct measure of disease/disability/injury rate or risk
Allows for hypothesis testing on the magnitude of the effect of the risk factor(s) on the outcome of the health-related event (disease/disability/injury)

VIII. Limitations of Prevalence Data in Public Health

A. Tends to produce biased picture of the health-related events such as disease, favoring the inclusion of chronic over acute diseases.

B. Cause and effect are measured simultaneously.

C. Cannot be used for causal inference.

D. Determined from one survey, whereas incidence requires at least two sets of observations (records/data) of the same subject.

IX. Types of Rates (Crude, Specific, Adjusted)

A. *Crude rates* are based on the actual number of events in a population over a given time period.

  1. Examples of crude rates are birth rate, infant mortality rate, fetal death rate, maternal mortality rate, etc.

B. Crude birth rate is computed by the basic formula Number of live births within a given period/Population size at the middle of that period $\times$ 1,000 population.

  1. *Vignettes*: Consider a population of Newcountry to be 280,000,000 during 1996, and the number of babies born was 4,500,000 during the same period.
  2. The crude birth rate will be Number of live births (A)/Population size (B) $\times$ 1,000. Substituting for A and B $\rightarrow$ 4,500,000/280,000,000 $\times$ 1,000 = 16.07 per 1,000.

Table 2-6 Crude Rates: Example and Basic Formula for Rate Estimation

Crude Rate	Formula	Interpretation
Birth rate	Number of live births within a given period/Population size at the middle of that period × 1,000 population	Projects population changes Affected by number of women of childbearing age
Infant mortality	Number of infant deaths among infants aged 0 to 365 days during the year/ Number of live births during the year × 1,000 live births	Used for international comparison Low rates reflect balanced health needs
Post-neonatal mortality rate	Number of infant deaths from 28 to 365 days after birth/Number of live births minus neonatal deaths × 1,000 live births	Low rates reflect environmental events, infectious disease control, and adequate nutrition

C. The rate is often incorrectly used to refer to proportions or ratios, as in these illustrations.

D. *Vignettes*: Consider a population of 200,000 people of whom 40 are diagnosed with pancreatic neoplasm (PN) in 2005, and during the same time period (2005), 36 died from pancreatic neoplasm. How will you calculate the mortality rate in 2005, and the case fatality rate in this population?

   1. Computation: (1) Mortality rate as a result of PN: 36/200,000 = 0.00018 (0.018%) or 18.0 per 100,000. (2) Case fatality as a result of PN: 36/40 = 0.9 (90%).

E. *Specific rates* refer to a particular subgroup of the population defined such as age, sex, social class, and race. Example of specific rate is age-specific rate.

F. Age-specific rate refers to the number of cases per age group of population during a specified time period.
   1. *Vignette*: Consider that in No-county during 2006, there were 1,100 deaths due to bronchial carcinoma (BC) among the 55–74 age group, and there were 35,000,000 persons in the same age group. What will be the age-specific bronchial carcinoma death rate in this age group?
   2. *Computation*: Using the formula Number of deaths (BC) among those aged 55–74 years (*A*)/Number of persons aged 55–74 years during 2006; (*B*) × 100,000. Substituting → $A/B \times 100{,}000$; $1{,}100/35{,}000{,}000 \times 100{,}000 = 3.14$ per 100,000.

G. *Adjusted rates* refers to summary measures of the rate of morbidity and mortality in a population in which statistical procedures have been applied to remove the effect of differences in the composition of the various populations such as age for the purpose of comparison.

H. Two methods of rates adjustment are most commonly used in public health:
   1. *Direct method* is used if age-specific death rates in a population to be standardized are known and a suitable standard population is available.
   2. *Indirect method* or standardized mortality ratios (SMR) is used when the age-specific death rates are unknown or unstable.

I. *Direct method*: (1) Multiply the age-specific rate by the number of persons. (2) Sum the expected number of deaths in each age group to determine the total number of expected deaths. (3) The age-adjusted rate is Total expected number of deaths/Number of deaths in the standardized or combined population, × 100,000.
   1. The result, the adjusted death rate, ensures that the observed differences in the death rates between the two populations compared are not due to age, gender, or sex.

2. *Vignettes*: Using Table 2.7, consider the age group in years, the age-specific death rates per 100,000 in Populations *X* and *Y*, and the number in the United States in 1998 (census population estimates). Determine which population has excess mortality.

Table 2-7 Age-Specific Mortality Rates for Populations *X* and *Y*

Age Group	(*A*) Population *X* (Age-specific rates per 100,000)	(*B*) Population *Y* (Age-specific rates per 100,000)	(*C*) U.S. Population (1998 Census estimate)	(*D*) (Expected death for population *X*)	(*E*) (Expected death for population *Y*)
< 5 years	149.19	181.40	18,989,257		
5–19	43.44	36.78	58,712,947		
20–24	165.97	178.23	100,919,429		
45–64	521.18	725.04	57,241,131		
> 65 years	4,011.94	4,517.68	34,385,239		
Total	417.91	1,060.94	270,248,003		

Source: Data from National Center for Health Statistics, Division of Data Services.

3. *Computation*: (1) Multiply *A* by *C* to obtain *D*, expected deaths for population *X*. (2) Multiply *B* and *C* to obtain *E*, expected death for population *Y*. (3) Obtain the age adjusted rate for population *X* by summing the total in column *D* and dividing by the total in column *C*, then multiplying by 100,000. (4) Repeat the steps in 3 for population *Y*. (5) Subtract the rate in *X* (702.56 per 100,000) from *Y* (815.15 per 100.000). The excess age-adjusted mortality rate is 112.6 per 100,000.

J. *Indirect age-adjusted rate* (SMR) is calculated by Observed number of deaths (A)/Expected number of deaths $(B) \times 100$.
   1. *Vignettes*: Consider the number of observed deaths in Notown from angina pectoris to be 1,200 during 2005. If the expected number of deaths is 2,000, what is the SMR?
   2. *Computation*: SMR $= A/B \times 100$. Substituting → 1,200/2,000 = 0.6 (60%).

X. Measures of Disease Comparison

A. *Absolute*
   1. Subtracted from one another.
   2. Provide information about public health impact of an exposure.

B. *Relative*
   1. Divided from one another.
   2. Provide information about the strength of the relationship between exposure (independent variable) and outcome (disease, disabilities, or injuries).

C. Absolute measures of comparison are risk difference, rate difference, incidence rate difference, cumulative incidence difference, and prevalence difference.

D. Relative measures of comparison are risk ratio, rate ratio, relative rate or relative risk, incidence rate ratio, cumulative incidence ratio, and prevalence ratio.

E. *Rate versus risk*
   1. Risk is the accumulated effect of rate occurring during some specified time period.
   2. Risk has no time dimension, and the reference population in risk is the population unaffected at the beginning of the period of observation.

F. *Attack rate* (AR), although not specifically a rate but a proportion, is the cumulative incidence of a disease during an outbreak or transient epidemic.

1. AR = Diseased (exposed and developed an illness)/Diseased and Nondiseased (all exposed to the suspected agent of contamination) × (multiplier [100]) during a time period.

G. *Secondary attack rate* (SAR) is the proportion of individuals exposed to the primary case (primary cases), who themselves develop the disease (secondary cases).
   1. SAR = Number of new cases in group − Initial case(s)/Number of susceptible persons in a group − Initial case(s).

H. *Vignette*: Consider data on primary and secondary attack from salmonella pathogen. Is this a rate or ratio?
   1. *Solution*: Because time is not involved in the denominator, this measure of disease is strictly not a rate but a risk (proportion).

Table 2-8 Measures of Comparison

Measure	Formula	Explanation
Rate or risk ratio	*RE/RU*, where *RE* = risk or rate in the exposed and *RU* = risk or rate in the unexposed	Measures the strength of association between exposure and the disease (outcome)
Attributable proportion among total population	(*RT* – *RU*)/*RT* × 100, where *RT* = incidence rate (IR), cumulative incidence (CI), or prevalence proportion (PP) in the total population and *RU* is the IR, CI, or PP in the unexposed population	Measures the excess proportion of disease in the total population, assuming the exposure is causal and implying that the proportion of a disease in a total population that will be eliminated if the exposure were eliminated

Table 2-8 Measures of Comparison *(continued)*

Measure	Formula	Explanation
Attributable proportion among the exposed	$(RE - RU)/RE \times 100$	Measures the proportion of disease among the exposed, assuming the exposure is causal and implying the proportion of disease among the exposed that will be eliminated if the exposure is eliminated
Population rate difference	$RT - RU$ or $RD \times PE$, where $RD =$ IR difference, CI difference, or PP difference; and $PE =$ proportion of population that is exposed, and $RD = RE - RU$	Measures excess rate or risk of a disease or outcome in the total population
Rate or risk difference	$RE - RU$	Measures rate or risk of disease or outcome among the exposed population
Attack rate	ND/TP, where $ND =$ number of people at risk in whom a certain outcome develops, and $TP =$ total number of people at risk	Compares the risk of outcome in groups with different exposure

XI. Sources of Epidemiologic Data

Table 2-9 Sources of Epidemiologic Data

Sources	Description
Vital statistics	Provides information for births, deaths, marriages, and divorces
U.S. Census	Provides information on complete counts of U.S. population every 10 years
	Types of information include race, sex, age, and marital status (all samples); and income, education level, housing, and occupation (representative samples)
National health interview survey	Provides data on major health problems, such as acute and chronic disease conditions, impairment and injuries, and utilization of the health services, such as dental care
	Useful in examining annual changes in disease and disabilities conditions
National health and nutrition examination survey (NHANES)	Provides information on the health and diet of the U.S. population based on home interview and nutritional examination
Behavioral risk factor surveillance system	Survey of random sample of U.S. population by phone interviews on behaviors affecting health and well-being (exercise, smoking, obesity, alcohol, automobile seat belts, and drinking and driving)
National notifiable diseases surveillance system	Provides information on most communicable diseases, including HIV/AIDS, botulism, gonorrhea, human and animal rabies, etc.

Table 2-9 Sources of Epidemiologic Data *(continued)*

Sources	Description
Surveillance, epidemiology, and end results program (SEER)	National Cancer Institute database that provides information on trends in cancer incidence, mortality, and survival Information includes patient demographics, primary cancer sites, pathology, first mode of therapy, and severity of the disease
World Health Statistics Annual	Provides information on international morbidity and mortality
Cancer Incidence of Five Continents	WHO's international agency for research and cancer that provides information on cancer incidence and mortality globally (estimated 170 cancer registries in 50 countries)
National occupational hazards survey and national occupational exposure survey	Provides data on workers exposed to chemical, physical, and biologic agents
Surveillance of AIDS and HIV infection	Provides information on HIV/AIDS incidence and prevalence, as well as cumulative incidence

XII. Epidemiologic Study Designs (Experimental and Observational)

A. Designs in epidemiologic investigations may be observational (the investigator does not manipulate the assignment of subjects) or experimental (subjects are randomized to the various arms of treatment or placebo).

B. Epidemiologic designs commonly used are *ecologic, case-control/comparison, cross-sectional* (prevalence), *cohort* (longitudinal), *retrospective cohort* (historical/nonconcurrent prospective study), *prospective cohort* (concurrent/concurrent prospective), and *experimental* (randomized trial).

C. The main goal of analytic design is to determine whether there is an association between the factors or characteristics and the development of a disease, disabilities, or injuries.

D. If association exists, design also allows one to derive appropriate inferences regarding a potential causal relationship.

E. Analysis could be at individual level as in cross-sectional study, case-control study, cohort study, and clinical trials.

F. Analysis could also be at the group level, for example, ecologic design. (Be conscious of ecologic fallacy, which claims that an association occurs at individual level when the analysis was performed at a group level.)

1. *Ecologic design*
    a. An observational epidemiologic study design.
    b. Examines the relationship between exposure and the outcome of interest (disease, disability, and injury) with population level rather than the individual level as a unit of data gathering and analysis.
    c. Correlation coefficient is the point estimate for the measure of association.
    d. Limitations include the inability to establish temporal sequence and the tendency to make cross-level inferences from group to individual (ecologic fallacy).

2. *Cross-sectional design*

Table 2-10 Cross-Sectional (Prevalence) Design: Description, Measure of Association, Strengths, and Limitations

Description

- Snapshots of a population at a single point in time.
- Defines a population and determines the presence or absence of exposure and the presence or absence of disease for each subject.

Measure of association

- Measure of the exposure prevalence in relation to disease, disability, or injury prevalence.
- Using a 2 × 2 table, the prevalence of the disease in the exposed: $a/a + b$; presence of the disease in subjects without exposure: $c/c + d$; prevalence of exposure in persons with the disease: $a/a + c$, and prevalence of exposure in subjects without disease: $b/b + d$.
- Prevalence risk/odds ratio: $a/a + b \,/\, c/c + d$; where $a =$ exposed and diseased, $b =$ exposed and non-diseased, $c =$ unexposed but diseased, and $d =$ unexposed and non-diseased.

Strengths and advantages

- Generalizability.
- Inexpensive.

Limitations

- Inability to assess temporal sequence between exposure and disease or health-related events if exposure changes over time (not possible to tell whether the exposure preceded the development of disease).
- Preponderance of prevalent cases of long duration.
- Healthy worker survival effects (association may be due to survival after the health-related event rather than with the risk of development of health-related event).

Table 2-10 Cross-Sectional (Prevalence) Design: Description, Measure of Association, Strengths, and Limitations *(continued)*

Vignettes

- Consider a study that is interested in the possible association between low serum lycopene level (exposure) and prostate cancer (disease). If the population is surveyed and the serum lycopene is determined for all subjects, perform prostate specific antigen (PSA) for prostate cancer, and both exposure and disease are determined at the same time.
  a. Could this constitute a cross-sectional design?
  b. Calculate the prevalence risk ratio if 20 of the 60 men with low serum lycopene level had prostate cancer while 10 of the 80 men with high serum lycopene level had prostate cancer.
- *Computing*: Prevalence risk ratio: $a/a + b / c/c + d$. Substituting → 20/80 / 10/90 = 0.25/0.11 = 2.27.

3. *Case-control or comparison design*

Table 2-11 Case-Control Design: Description, Measure of Association, Strengths, and Limitations

Description

- Method of sampling a population in which epidemiologists (investigators) identify and enroll cases of disease or health-related event and a sample of the source population that produced the cases.
- Hallmark of case-control study (CCS) is that it begins with the disease (cases) and compares them to people without disease (control).
- Compares a group of individuals who have experienced the outcome (health-related event) under study (cases) with a group who have not (control or comparison).

Table 2-11 Case-Control Design: Description, Measure of Association, Strengths, and Limitations *(continued)*

- Cases are identified (formulation of a disease or case definition) as whether they belong to exposed or unexposed group (cohort), whereas the control is sampled from the source population.
- The control group is used to estimate the distribution of the exposure in the source population; control must be sampled independently of the exposure status.
- Variant designs:
  - *Case-crossover*, a design where cases serve as their own controls; is appropriate in settings in which the risk of the outcome is increased for only a brief time following exposure (typical exposure is something that varies from time to time within an individual).
  - Uses the previous experience of the cases as a substitute for control series to estimate the person-time distribution in the source population.
  - *Nested case-control*, a hybrid design where new case controls are derived from a cohort study (nested) of the original design.
  - *Case-cohort*, study in which every person in the source population has the same chance of being included as a control, regardless of the time contributed by that person to the person-time experience of the cohort.

Measure of association

- Using a 2×2 table, the sample of all available cases $= (a + c)$, and independently, a sample of unaffected subjects (comparison/control) $= (b + d)$.
- The primary measure of association is odds ratio or relative odds, which is simply the cross-products ratio.
- Odds ratio (OR) is calculated by multiplying the number opposite it on the diagonal of the 2×2 table, and this result is then divided by the two other numbers multiplied together (cross-products ratio).
- $OR = (a/b) / (c/d) \rightarrow ad/bc$ (cross products).
- *Odds concept*: The odds that the case was exposed: a/c, whereas the odds that a control was exposed: b/d. The odds ratio is simply the ratio that the cases were exposed to the odds that the controls were exposed: a/c

Table 2-11 Case-Control Design: Description, Measure of Association, Strengths, and Limitations *(continued)*

divided by *b/d*. Therefore OR = (product of diseased people exposed and non-diseased people unexposed) *ad*/(product of non-diseased people exposed and diseased people unexposed) *bc* → OR = *ad/bc*.

Strengths and advantages

- Efficient for rare diseases (desirable design).
- Efficient for diseases with long induction and latent periods.
- Adequate for evaluating multiple exposures in relation to a disease (desirable when little is known about exposure variables in a given disease).
- Rapid and inexpensive relative to prospective cohort design.

Limitations

- Recall and selection bias. Recall bias due to the retrospective nature of the design.
- Difficult to assess temporal sequence between exposure and disease or health-related events if exposure changes over time.
- Information bias and poor information on exposure (retrospective nature of the design).
- Inefficient for rare exposure.

Vignettes

- Consider a study that is interested in the possible association between smoking (exposure) and coronary heart disease [CHD] (disease). If the investigators begin with 400 people with CHD (cases) and compare them with 800 controls (people without CHD), is this a case-control investigation? Suppose 224 of the 400 cases were smokers and 176 were nonsmokers. Of the 800 controls, 352 were smokers and 448 were nonsmokers.
    a. What is the measure of association in this investigation, and how could this be calculated?
- *Computing*: The exposure odds ratio: *ad/bc*. Substituting → 224 × 448 / 176 × 352 = 1.62. This result indicates that individuals with smoking history had a 62% increased risk of experiencing CHD compared to those with no history of smoking.

a. Note: (1) Because the two groups are sampled separately, rates of disease, disabilities, or injuries in the exposed or unexposed groups cannot be calculated, nor can relative risk be measured directly. However, the odds ratio can be computed, which is the primary measure of association in case-control design. (2) Because of the sampling used, the total number exposed is not $a + b$, and the risk in exposed subjects is not $a/(a + b)$.

b. Nested case control is advantageous to the classic case-control in that (1) it minimizes and eliminates recall bias; (2) it ensures or reduces temporal sequence, thus making it easy to determine whether the exposure preceded the disease; and (3) it is relatively inexpensive and rapid, compared to prospective cohort design.

c. Nested case control is limited in that the non-diseased may not be fully representative of the original cohort due to loss to follow-up or death.

d. Odds ratio is a good estimate of relative risk, except when the outcome is very frequent (high prevalence).

e. *Odds and probability (case-control versus cohort design)*: Odds differs from probability (P), but is related by: Odds = P /1 – P. For example, if the probability of diseased being exposed is 80% (0.8), the odds of diseased being exposed are 4.0, which is 80/20 (P/1 – P).

   1. In a cohort design, the probability that the exposed will develop a disease is $a/a + b$ and the odds that a disease will develop in the exposed is a/b (P/1 – P). The probability that the disease will develop in unexposed is $c/c + d$, similarly, the odds of disease developing in unexposed is c/d (P/1 – P).
   2. The odds ratio (*incidence rate ratio*) in cohort design *is* a/b / c/d = ad/bc, which is the odds that an exposed person develops a disease divided by the odds that a non-exposed person develops disease.

4. *Cohort design*

Table 2-12 Cohort Design: Description, Measure of Association, Strengths, and Limitations

Description

- Design that represents a group of individuals who are followed over a period of time for the occurrence of a specific disease(s), disability, or injury.
- Typically comprises two cohorts, namely, exposed and unexposed.
- The purpose of follow-up is to measure the occurrence of the health-related event(s), with the aim of comparing the specific disease(s), disability, or injury rates for two or more cohorts.
- Two cohorts are commonly followed in epidemiology: (1) *closed* (fixed membership—allows no addition of individual once follow up begins), example, randomized clinical trial, and (2) *open* (dynamic cohort that can take new members as time passes), example, state cancer registries that comprises the state residents, and is dynamic because new residents may be added to the registry.
- The study group is the exposed, while the comparison is the unexposed.

Measure of association

- Risk or incidence can be estimated from a closed cohort. Please note that the computation of risk is complicated by competing risk—the removal of some subjects from the population at risk before they have experienced the entire follow-up period.
- Risk can be estimated directly if there is (1) a short follow-up period ($<$ 30 days) or (2) a small competing risk (very few or no deaths).
- Under this assumption (short follow-up period and no competing risk), risk is estimated by dividing the number of new health-related events by the total number of people being followed (population at risk) in the closed cohort.
- Incidence rate (IR) calculation is the appropriate measure and a more reliable estimate if the cohort is dynamic. Therefore, one must take into account the amount of time each person contributes as a member of the population at risk in addressing competing risk in the dynamic as well as close cohort that is designated with a long follow-up period and competing risks.

Table 2-12 Cohort Design: Description, Measure of Association, Strengths, and Limitations *(continued)*

- IR is computed by dividing the number of new cases (incident cases) by the amount of person-time experienced by the population at risk.
- *Computation*: Relative risk (RR) = $a/a + b$ (incidence in the exposed) / c/c + d (incidence in the unexposed). Where the denominator is the person-time, the RR represents the incidence rate (IR) or incidence density (ID).
- *RR interpretation*: (1) RR = 1.0 (no association—null), (2) RR > 1.0 (positive association—predisposing/possibly causal), or (3) RR < 1.0 (negative association—protective).

Strengths and advantages

- Efficient for rare exposure.
- Establishes a clear temporal relationship between exposure and the outcome of interest (prospective design).
- Particularly efficient for diseases with long induction and latent periods (retrospective design).
- Produces a direct measure of risk or incidence of disease.
- Produces reliable information on exposures, especially prospective designs.
- Appropriate in assessing multiple effects of an exposure.
- Feasible relative to experimental design when ethical consideration precludes such conduct (less vulnerable to ethical restrictions of randomized clinical trials).

Limitations

- Relatively expensive compared to case-control or cross-sectional design.
- Takes long time to conduct, (loss to follow-up, change of exposure over time → exposure misclassification → attenuation of the point estimate [RR]).
- Inefficient for diseases with long induction and latent periods (prospective design).
- Inefficient for rare outcomes (prospective design).

Table 2-12 Cohort Design: Description, Measure of Association, Strengths, and Limitations *(continued)*

- Vulnerable to information and other types of bias (selection, misclassification)—retrospective design.
- Minimal information on exposure and some key variables, restricting controlling for confounders due to unmeasured confounding → biased point estimate (retrospective design).

Vignettes

- Consider a cohort study to compare the mortality rate of myocardial infarction (MI) in men with sedentary work (exposed group) to men with physically active work (unexposed). If in the exposed, there were 18,000 person man-years of observation and 63 deaths; whereas the unexposed had 12,000 man-years of observation and 22 deaths:
  a. What will the mortality rate be in each cohort?
  b. What is the relative risk/incidence density of dying, comparing these two groups?
  c. What is the attributable risk of sedentary work?
  d. What is the attributable benefit of physical activity?
  e. If we assume that MI is associated with the mortality in this cohort (causality), what proportion of disease in the higher risk group is potentially preventable?

Computation

- (a) *Mortality rate* in each cohort (1) Exposed group → Number of deaths among those in the sedentary group (exposed) / Person-time experience → 63/18,000 = 0.0035 (multiplier − 100,000) → 0.0035 × 100,000 = 350 deaths per 100,000 man-years; (2) Using the same basic formula in (1) and substituting: 22/12,000 → 0.0018 (multiplier − 100,000) → 0.0018 × 100,000 = 183 deaths per 100,000 man-years.
- (b) *Relative risk*: Risk in the exposed/ Risk in the unexposed → 350/183 per 100,000 man-years = 1.91.
- (c) *Attributable risk* (risk difference) of sedentary work: Risk in the exposed − Risk in the unexposed → 350 − 183 deaths per 100,000 →167 deaths per 100,000 man-years.

Table 2-12 Cohort Design: Description, Measure of Association, Strengths, and Limitations *(continued)*

- (d) *Attributable benefit* of physical activity simply implies the risk difference → 167 deaths per 100,000.
- (e) *Attributable proportion* in the exposed = Attributable risk (*A*)/Total risk in the exposed (*B*). Also, (RR -1) / (RR).
- *Substituting*: *A/B* = 167/350 per 100,000 man-years → 47.7%. Thus, the preventable proportion as a result of eliminating sedentary lifestyle in the exposed group will be 47.7% of deaths due to MI in this group.

a. *Desirability of cohort designs*
   1. Use cohort design (prospective) when: (a) multiple effects of exposure are assessed or (b) exposure is rare.
   2. Use cohort design (retrospective) when (a) outcome of interest has long induction period, (b) outcome of interest has a long latent period, or (c) outcome is rare.

b. *Types of cohort designs*:
   1. *Prospective*: Study subjects are selected on the basis of exposure and followed over time.
   2. *Retrospective*: Both the exposure and outcome of interest have already occurred prior to the commencement of study.
   3. *Ambidirectional*: Cohort study with both prospective and retrospective components.

5. *Experimental design*

Table 2-13 Experimental Designs: Description, Measure of Association, Strengths, and Limitations

Description

- Nonobservational and involves random assignment of subjects to treatment and control groups.
- Best design of studying new interventions on individual or community basis.
- Prospective in time relationship.
- Gold standard of epidemiologic investigation when feasible; allows randomized double-blinded placebo-control assessment.

Measure of association

- Same as prospective cohort study (relative risk, odds ratio, hazard ratio).
- Unlike prospective cohort, the analysis to yield the point estimate could be:
  (a) *Intent-to-treat analysis* (data on the effectiveness of treatment under everyday practice condition; all randomized subjects whether or not there is an assurance on treatment compliance).
  (b) *Efficacy analysis* (data on treatment effects under ideal condition).

Strengths and advantages

- Randomization—most appropriate way to control confounding.
- Double blinded—most appropriate way to control bias.
- Provides direct measure of association for benefits or risk (relative risk, risk ratio, hazard ratio).

Limitations

- Loss to follow-up (prospective), especially in long-term trials involving many years of follow-up.
- Generalizability—efficacy treatment may not necessarily translate to effectiveness of the treatment in real-world situations (community settings).
- Ethical consideration—patients cannot be assigned to exposure with known adverse effects, such as tobacco ingestion.

Table 2-13 Experimental Designs: Description, Measure of Association, Strengths, and Limitations *(continued)*

Vignette (1)

- Consider a clinical trial of 2,000 subjects (close cohort) with angina pectoris (AP) of whom half (1,000, intervention/treatment) received Nitroglycerin-G2 (new drug) and the other half (1,000, control) received the standard therapy (Nitroglycerin). After 5 years of follow-up, 200 deaths were reported in the intervention group and 350 from the control. If we assume non-differential loss to follow-up or no loss in the two arms, what is the relative mortality associated with the new drug? What is your interpretation of the result?
- *Computation*: (1) Mortality rate in the intervention = Number of deaths/Population at risk. Substituting → 200/1,000 = 0.2 (20%). (2) Mortality rate in the control = Number of deaths (control group)/Population at risk (control group). Substituting → 350/1,000 = 0.35 (35%). (3) Relative mortality associated with the new drug = Rate in the intervention group/Rate in the control group. Substituting → 0.2/0.35 = 0.57.
- *Interpretation*: Relative risk less than 1.0 is indicative of the protective effect of the new drug with respect to mortality in the intervention population compared to the control.

Vignette (2)

- Consider a clinical trial of Bacillus Calmette-Guerin (BCG) vaccination in which 556 children were vaccinated and 8 died and 528 were not (control) and 8 died. Assuming this was a randomized clinical trial, what is the relative risk of dying? Is the vaccine protective against dying compared with the placebo (control)?
- *Computation*: (1) Mortality rate in the vaccinated = Number of deaths in the vaccinated group/Population at risk (vaccinated children). Substituting → 8/556 = 0.014 (1.44%). (2) Mortality rate in the control group = Number of deaths in the control group/Population at risk (control). Substituting → 8/528 = 0.015 (1.51%). Relative risk = Rate in the vaccinated children/rate in the control. Substituting → 1.44/1.51 = 0.95.
- *Interpretation*: The relative risk less than 1.0 (null − no association) is indicative of the benefit of the vaccine in decreasing mortality in the vaccinated group compared with the control.

a. *Types of experimental trial*: (1) cross-over (each group receives all treatment but not simultaneously), (2) parallel (each group receives one treatment but treatments are administered concurrently), (3) simple (each group receives only one treatment), (4) factorial (each group receives two or more treatments), (5) community, (6) individual, (7) preventive, and (8) therapeutic.
b. *Double blinded*: Neither the experimenter nor the study subjects have knowledge of the intervention assignment.
c. *Placebo control*: The control group is given an inactive treatment (water pill/nondrug), which resembles the intervention drug.

6. *Meta-analytic design (quantitative systematic review)*
   a. Method of combining the results from a number of studies of similar design to produce an overall estimate of effect, which incorporates the information provided by all the studies.
      1. Popular method of critically assessing the value of evidence used to support health interventions—evidence-based medicine, quantitative evidence synthesis (QES).
      2. Useful in answering research questions whenever an investigation of a particular research subject presents with conflicting or contradictory results. For example, some research groups may report a statistically significant difference in the use of anti-androgen in prolonging survival of men treated for loco-regional prostate cancer while other groups report no statistically significant difference.
      3. A method of summarizing, integrating, and interpreting research studies that produces quantitative findings.
      4. A technique of encoding and analyzing the statistics that summarize research findings.

b. If full datasets of studies of interest are available, a pool analysis is the preferred method.

c. Because meta-analysis focuses on the aggregation and comparison of findings of different research studies, meaningful comparability is required. For example, studies assessing the association between selenium intake and prostate cancer can be compared with meta-analytic design using prospective cohort or case-control studies but not mixed, given the differences in the point estimates generated by these two designs. Likewise, observational and experimental cannot be mixed in meta-analytic designs but can be compared separately.

d. Meta-analysis represents each study's findings in the form of effect sizes or point estimates. An effect size encodes the quantitative information from each relevant study's findings. Studies that produce bivariate correlations cannot be combined with those that compared groups of subjects on the mean values of the dependent variables.

e. *Methodology*: This involves (1) defining the research question, (2) defining the criteria for studies to be included, (3) identifying and retrieving the studies that meet the inclusion criteria, (4) abstracting information, (5) analyzing statistics (fixed effect or random-effect analysis), and (6) reporting results.

f. *Statistical/analytic methods*: *Fixed and random effect models.*

g. *Heterogeneity test*: Tests whether the overall summary estimate is an adequate representation of the dataset; compares each of the individual study results with the summary estimate; examines the differences between the studies.

   1. Based on weighted average of the difference of the results of each study and the summary estimate of the effect.

2. If there is significant heterogeneity, the analysis may be repeated after excluding the studies that are particularly divergent.
3. The heterogeneity statistics produce a χ^2 value for each individual study, based on the comparison of that study's result to the summary result.

h. *Fixed effects model*:
   1. Mantel–Haenszel: Attempts to derive the most useful summary estimate of effect from the data given all the studies included in the analysis.
      a. Similar to analysis of stratified data, where the stratification variable is the individual study.
   2. Peto: Utilizes a 2 × 2 table for the observed and expected, and the chi square value is obtained by $(O_i - E_i)$, and the variance of the expected (V_i) calculated.

i. *Random effects model:*
   1. Assumes that the studies that have been included are a representative sample of a hypothetical larger population of studies.
   2. Where there is no heterogeneity between studies, the fixed effect and random effects model yield the same result.
      a. But where there is heterogeneity, the random effects model may give a substantially different result.
   3. The most widely used random effects models is the DerSimonian–Laird method.
      a. This method weights the inverse of a combination of within-study variation and between-study variation; as this variance will be larger, the confidence interval of summary measure of effect will be wider.

j. With substantial between-study variance (heterogeneity), the DerSimonian–Laird method gives relatively more weight to the smaller studies.

Table 2-14 Advantages and Disadvantages of Meta-analysis

Advantages

- Utilizes structured research technique to summarize and analyze a body of research studies.
- Represents key study findings, that is, more differentiated from the conventional review process, that rely on qualitative summaries.
- Capable of finding effects or associations that are obscured in qualitative reviews.
- Provides organized and structured way of handling information from a large number of study findings under review.
- Homogeneity test, which indicates if a grouping of effect sizes are from different studies, shows more variation than would be expected from sampling error alone.
- Capable of performing meta-regression that is not feasible from other types of review.

Disadvantages

- Time consuming and specialized skills.
- Methodological issues—study mixing, different effect sizes, or measure of effect.
- Publication bias.
- Cannot overcome limitations of the individual studies that make up the sample size (k).

XIII. Study Validity (Bias, Confounding, Random Error)

A. *Validity* (internal validity) refers to lack of bias and confounding in the design of an epidemiologic study.

B. *External validity* refers to the generalization of the findings from a study to a larger population different from the population that was sampled.

1. External validity cannot be established without internal validity in the first place.

C. *Bias* is a systematic error that occurs as a result of the investigator's design or conduct of the study that eventually results in inaccurate assessment of the association between the exposure and the outcome of interest.

D. *Types of bias*: (1) recall bias (commonly encountered in case-control study) refers to inability to remember information regarding exposure, especially among the control resulting in misclassification bias; (2) misclassification bias (errors or mistakes in data acquisition that result in the wrong grouping of study subjects); (3) information bias (record abstraction, interviewing, surrogate interviews, recall bias, surveillance, reporting); and (4) selection bias.

E. *Surveillance bias*: Because populations with disease are more closely monitored compared with those who do not have the disease, disease ascertainment may be better in the monitored population and may introduce surveillance bias (monitoring of one population [diseased] more than the other [disease-free]). This bias may lead to erroneous estimation of the effect of the disease in the monitored population, thus inflating the point estimate (RR, OR).

F. *Controlling/minimizing bias*: (1) Accurate definition of items, (2) methods of measurement, (3) standardization of procedures, and (4) quality control of data collection and processing.

G. *Confounding* refers to the influence or effect of an extraneous factor(s) on the relationship or associations between the exposure and the outcome of interest.

1. Occurs when the effects of the exposure are mixed together with the effect of another variable, leading to a bias.
2. If exposure X causes disease Y, Z is a confounder if Z is a known risk factor for disease Y, and Z is associated with X, but Z is not a result of exposure X.
3. *Vignette*: Consider a study to assess the association between coffee drinking (X) and pancreatic cancer risk (Y). The exposure variable is coffee drinking, and coffee drinking is known to be associated with cigarette smoking (Z).

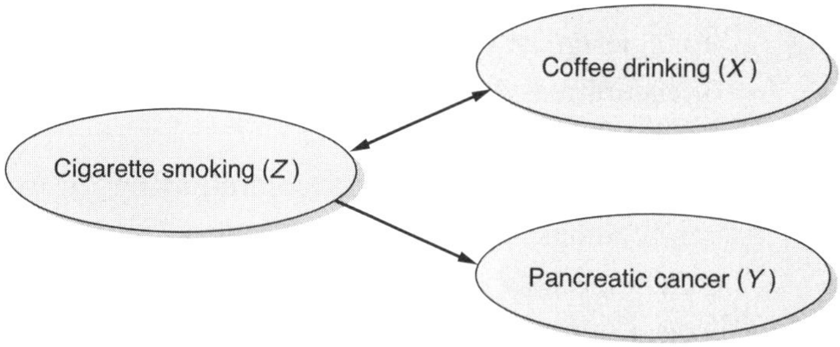

Figure 2-1 Confounding (illustrating the two associations that are necessary for it to occur).

Likewise, cigarette smoking is a known risk factor for pancreatic cancer. If causal association is observed between coffee drinking and pancreatic cancer, this might be due to the confounding effect of smoking. Therefore, to be confounding, smoking must be a risk factor for pancreatic cancer and be associated with coffee drinking.

If a causal association such as $X \rightarrow Y$ occurs, then this causal relationship may be due to Z (confounder).

H. Confounding per se is not a bias.

I. *Controlling for confounding* is a method of producing an unconfounded effect (point) estimate: (1) During the design phase of the study → (a) restriction, (b) matching, (c) randomization. (2) During analysis phase of the study→ (a) restriction, (b) stratification (stratified analysis), (c) multivariable method (analysis).

J. Random error refers to unsystematic errors that arise from an unforeseeable and unpredictable process, such as a mistake in assessing the exposure and disease, and sampling variability (unrepresentative sample, or chance).

K. Precision is the lack of random error.

1. Precision, and hence reduction in random error, may be reduced by (a) increasing the sample size, (b) repeating measurement within a study, and (c) utilizing an efficient study design in order to maximize the amount of information obtained.

2. Precision (lack of random error) may be influenced by (a) sampling, (b) hypothesis testing and p values, (c) confidence intervals estimation, (d) random variable probability distribution, and (e) sample size and power estimation.

L. Systematic error may be present in a study despite absence or reduction in random error (study may be precise but findings are inaccurate).

M. *Interaction* is said to occur when the incidence rate of a disease or outcome in the presence of two or more risk factors differs from the incidence rate expected to result from their individual effect. This rate may be greater than what is expected (synergism) or less than what is expected (antagonism).

N. Like effect measure modifier, interaction is said to occur if there is a difference in the strata-specific risk point estimate (RR, OR) on the basis of the third variable.

O. *Additive model*: Occurs in association of effect if the effect of one exposure is added to the effect of the other (e.g., if those with neither exposure have an incidence of 2.0). In those with smoking history, the incidence is 8.0, and 16.0 in those with smoking history and heavy alcohol consumption.

1. The additive model assumes that the incidence will be X in those with both types of risk. What is X? X is 22. Because smoking adds 6.0 to those with no risk, it will be expected to add 6.0 to those with alcohol drinking history.
2. Additive model is not accurate in describing the effect of exposure to two independent factors in disease causation.

P. *Multiplicative model*: Appropriate model for describing the effects of two independent factors or exposures in disease causation (e.g., if absence of neither exposure has an incidence of 2.0, and those exposed to cigarette smoking have an incidence of 8.0, while those exposed to heavy alcohol consumption have an incidence of 16.0).

1. The multiplicative model assumes that the incidence will be Y in those with both risks. What is Y? Y is 64. Because smoking

multiplies the risk by 4 times in the absence of alcohol, we also expect it to multiply the risk in alcohol users by 4 times (16×4). If so, the effect of exposure to both smoking and alcohol will be $16 \times 4 = 64$.

Q. Effect measure modifier or effect modification (heterogeneity of effect) refers to the strength of association between exposure and the disease that differs according to level of another variable (effect modifier). For example, age is a modifier in the association between ethnicity and hypertension. Differences are not observed between black and white men under the age of 35 with respect to hypertension incidence. After age 35, incidence tends to be 2 to 3 times higher in blacks relative to whites of the same age.

R. Biologically, an effect measure modifier is the third variable that is not a confounding but enters into a causal pathway between the exposure and the disease of interest. For example, the relationship between lung cancer and cigarette smoking is modified by asbestos, because asbestos exposure has been known to increase the risk of dying by 92 times among smokers, whereas the risk of dying from lung cancer among those exposed to asbestos only is 10-fold. Another example is the modifying effect of cigarette smoking and obesity on the association between oral contraceptives and myocardial infarction in women.

S. Effect measure modifier and confounding similarities:
   1. Both confounding and effect measure modifiers involve a third variable as well as is assessed or evaluated by performing stratified analysis.

T. Effect measure modifier versus confounding:
   1. In confounding, one is interested in knowing whether the crude measure of association (unadjusted point estimate) changes (distorted) and whether the stratum-specific and adjusted summary estimate differ from the crude or unadjusted estimate.

2. In effect measure modification, one is interested in finding out if the association differs according to the third variable (the difference in stratum-specific estimate from one another).

U. *Vignette*: Consider a case-control study of the effect of lycopene on prostate cancer stratified by body mass index (BMI) (normal versus overweight). The stratum-specific odds ratio for men with abnormal BMI ≥ 24.99 kg/m^2 $= 2.2$ and the stratum-specific odds ratio for men with normal BMI (< 24.99 kg/m^2) $= 1.0$. Does this illustration indicate the presence of effect modifier or confounding by BMI?

V. *Solution*: Because the stratum-specific odds ratio differs between men with normal and abnormal BMI, BMI is an effect measure modifier between lycopene and prostate cancer in men.
   1. In this example, the BMI needs to be described or explained in the causal pathway of prostate cancer and does not need to be adjusted for since it is not a confounding.

W. Can the same variable (gender) be an effect measure modifier and confounding in the same setting (simultaneously)?
   1. Explore this possibility using the combined odds ratio and stratum specific odds ratio illustration.

XIV. Epidemiologic Causal Inference

A. Epidemiologic investigation is concerned with association as well as causal association.

B. Simply, *cause* refers to whatever produces an effect (result, outcome, response variable).

C. Cause may be understood as a factor if its operation increases the frequency of an event (outcome, result).

D. Cause is also described as an event, condition, or characteristics that preceded a health-related event and without which the event would not have occurred at all or would not have occurred until some later time.

E. Causal inference in epidemiology involves two steps: (1) valid result—internal validity of the study (association that is not as a result of bias, confounding, and random error) and (2) assessing whether the exposure actually caused the effect (outcome, result).

F. Causal relationship may be:
   1. Necessary and sufficient (*necessary* if the outcome occurs only if the causal factor operated and *sufficient* if the operation of the causal factor *always* results in the outcome).
   2. Necessary but not sufficient.
   3. Sufficient but not necessary.
   4. Neither sufficient nor necessary, implying that the operation of the causal factor increases the frequency of the causal factor, but the outcome does not always result and the outcome can occur without the operation of the causal factor.

Table 2-15 Bradford Hill's Criteria for Causal Inference

Criteria	Explanation
Temporality	The cause must precede the outcome (disease) Complete consensus among investigators and most relevant criterion Easily established in prospective studies
Strength of association	Measured by relative risk or odds ratio Larger relative risk or odds ratio is more indicative of a stronger association
Dose-response (biologic gradient)	Effect increases as the exposure level increases
Consistency of association	Association is most likely to be causal if observed repeatedly by different persons, in different places, circumstances, and time
Plausibility	Coherency with the current body of knowledge (existence of biologic or social model to explain the association

Table 2-15 Bradford Hill's Criteria for Causal Inference *(cont.)*

Criteria	Explanation
Coherence	Cause and effect interpretation of the data should not seriously conflict with generally known facts of the natural history and the biology of the disease
Experiment	If exposure causes a disease, the disease is expected to decline when the exposure is reduced or eliminated
Analogy	Similarities between the observed association and other associations
Specificity	A cause should lead to a single effect and vice versa An association is specific when a certain exposure is associated with only one disease

G. *Rothman's sufficient: component cause model (causal pies)*
   1. Sufficient cause—complete causal mechanisms that inevitably produces disease.
   2. Component cause—each participating factor in a sufficient cause.
   3. Necessary cause—a causal component that is a member of every sufficient cause.
   4. The causal pies model indicates that a sufficient cause is not a single factor but rather a minimal set of factors that unavoidably produce disease, implying that the termination of the action of a single causal component blocks the completion of a sufficient cause, thus preventing disease occurrence by that pathway.

H. *Vignette 1*: Consider an epidemiologic investigation conducted to assess the association between exposure to sulfur and brain tumor in children. If the investigator wishes to compare the findings in this study with other evidence, which criteria according to Bradford Hill might be worth considering, and what sort of study design may provide a more valid and reliable comparison?

1. *Solution*: Evidence from one study may be compared with another in terms of Hill's criteria of consistency, plausibility, coherence, and specificity. The design most appropriate will be prospective.

I. *Vignette 2*: Consider an investigator who wishes to examine published studies on the evidence of estrogen replacement therapy in post-menopausal breast cancer. If he wishes to examine the features consistent with causation using Bradford Hill criteria, which features should be taken into consideration?

1. *Solution*: Bradford Hill's features consistent with causation are (a) temporal sequence, (b) strength of association, (c) dose response, (d) consistency, and (e) specificity.

J. *Vignette 3*: Consider an investigation of epidemiologic causal inference that attempts to examine the study validity prior to assessing whether the exposure actually led to the disease. Which aspects of the study must s/he consider in order to determine if the observed result was valid?

1. *Solution*: The first step in epidemiologic causal inference is to illustrate that the result was not due to (a) systematic error (bias), (b) confounding, or (c) random error.

REVIEW QUESTIONS (MULTIPLE CHOICE)

Directions: Each of the following questions contains multiple suggested responses. Select the *one best* response to each question.

1. Epidemiology could be defined as the study of distribution, determinants, and control of health-related states or events in the specified population and the application of this study to control health problems. As an epidemiologist, if required to fulfill the "distribution" and "determinant" components of this definition, what will this entail?

a. Public health infrastructure
b. Information, behavior, and health skills development
c. Information dissemination to the population at risk
d. Frequency, patterns, and causes of health-related events
e. Prevention of health-related events

2. In a survey conducted to examine the prevalence of two diseases, *X* and *Y*, in a specific population, the investigators found that the prevalence of disease *X* was higher than the prevalence of disease *Y*. If the incidence and seasonal pattern of both diseases are similar, which of these statements are consistent with this observation?

a. Patients die quickly from disease *Y* but not disease *X*
b. Patients die quickly from disease *X* but not disease *Y*
c. Patients recover more quickly from disease *Y* than from disease *X*
d. Patients recover more quickly from disease *X* than from disease *Y*
e. a and c only

3. The approach to epidemiology can be described as descriptive, which involves the analysis of disease, disability, and injury patterns by person, place, and time. During the summer of 2006, there was an outbreak of bacterial meningitis in Nocity, Illinois. If you are appointed to investigate this epidemic using a descriptive epidemiologic approach, what are the main reasons for describing this outbreak by person, place, and time?

a. To assess the health status of the Nocity population
b. To generate a hypothesis about the causal factors (causative pathogen/s) for this epidemic
c. To plan and evaluate the public health programs to manage this epidemic
d. a and c only
e. All of the above

4. During the third week of January 2006, 80 persons in Newtown of a population of 450 attended a wedding ceremony, which included a meal prepared by several of the participants. Within 2 days, 35 of the participants became ill with salmonellosis. Estimate the attack rate among the participants.

a. 7.7/100
b. 43.75/100
c. 17.7/100
d. 21.2/100
e. None of the above

5. In a small community of 1,000 households with a population of 5,000 people, 150 persons were affected with E. Coli gastroenteritis in 100 households. A total of 500 persons lived in the 100 affected households. If each household had only one primary case, estimate the secondary attack rate.

a. 12.5%
b. 30.0%
c. 10.0%
d. 25.0%
e. 37.5%

6. The accompanying table shows the number of persons who did and did not eat egg salad and those who did and did not develop group A streptococci. Using this information, estimate the relative risk of Group A streptococci in the exposed.

Exposure	Group A Streptococci	Non-Group A Streptococci	Total
Egg salad	46	22	68
Non-egg salad	13	46	59
Total	59	68	127

a. 0.68
b. 3.07
c. 0.22
d. 7.39
e. 0.88

7. In the Framingham Heart Study (FHS), the residents of the state of Massachusetts have been followed since the1950s to identify occurrence (heart disease) and risk factors for heart disease. This study identified high blood pressure, hyperlipidemia, stress, and physical inactivates as risk factors in heart disease. This dynamic cohort now involves the grandchildren of the original cohort. Which of the following study designs represent this study?

a. Case cross-over
b. Ambi-directional cohort
c. Retrospective cohort
d. Case control
e. None of the above

8. A study was conducted in which men (15–49 years) with testicular neoplasm and a comparable group of men (15–49 years) without testicular neoplasm were asked about their prior use of steroidal anti-inflammatory drugs. If you assume that the subjects were selected on the basis of disease and not exposure, and the risk as a measure of association is not directly estimated but obtained as odds ratio, this is an example of which type of design(s)?

a. Experimental
b. Observational
c. Cohort
d. Case control
e. b and d only

9. Epidemiologic designs are largely observational. Often, the critical issue restricting the conduct of experimental, clinical, or intervention trial is the ethical consideration such as assigning humans to a known carcinogen (e.g., nicotine). Which of the following statements illustrate(s) the distinction between the two designs?

a. Investigator is "blinded" (prevented from knowing the subjects' true exposure status until the end of the study) in an experimental study but not in an observational study
b. Investigator controls the subject's outcome in an experimental study but not in an observational study
c. Investigator controls the subject's exposure in an experimental study but not in an observational study
d. Experimental studies are conducted with animals; observational studies are conducted with humans
e. a and c only

10. Confounding is the mixing effect of an extraneous variable in the association between the predictor (independent variable) and outcome (dependent variable). A study was conducted to examine the association between pancreatic cancer and coffee drinking. If a third variable, cigarette smoking, is assumed to be a confounder in this association, which of the following features will qualify smoking as a confounder in this association?

a. Smoking is associated with coffee drinking in the population that produced the cases
b. Smoking is an independent cause or predictor of pancreatic cancer
c. Smoking is not an intermediate step in the causal pathway between coffee drinking and pancreatic cancer
d. a and c only
e. All of the above

11. Clinicians may examine men who are diabetic more often or more thoroughly than men who are not. If this observation is accurate, and if an association is observed between erectile dysfunction (ED) and diabetes mellitus in men, the association may be due to which of the following bias?

a. Misclassification bias
b. Recall bias
c. Surveillance bias
d. Interviewer bias
e. None of the above

Questions 12 & 13. A cohort study was conducted to assess the association between incidence of diabetes mellitus type II and exercise, where obesity is assumed to be a confounding factor. Using the accompanying table, attempt the following questions.

Exercise Level	DM (Type II)	Person-years	Incidence/ 100,000
All subjects (n = 8,000 person-years)			
Low	105	4,000	
High	25	4,000	6.25
Relative Risk			
BMI (> 24.99 kg/m^2) (n = 4,000 person-years)			
Low	90	3,000	30.0
High	10	1,000	
Relative risk			
BMI (< 24.99 kg/m2) (n = 4,000 person-years)			
Low	15	1,000	
High	15	3,000	5.0
Relative risk			

12. What is the relative risk for low exercise compared with high exercise in all subjects in the study?

a. 3.0
b. 2.3
c. 4.2
d. 2.4
e. Cannot be estimated from the information provided

13. If the relative risk in all subjects differs from the relative risk in the subjects stratified by BMI, which of the following statements may explain this observation?

a. BMI itself is a factor in type II DM
b. BMI is related to exercise
c. BMI is a confounder
d. All of the above
e. None of the above

14. The incidence rate of chronic obstructive pulmonary disease (COPD) in those who smoke is 400 per 10,000 person-years; in those who are exposed to air pollution, 200; and in those with neither exposure, 40. Estimate the incidence rate in those with both exposures, assuming an additive model.

a. 560 per 10,000 person-years
b. 640 per 10,000 person-years
c. 600 per 10,000 person-years
d. 240 per 10,000 person-years
e. 440 per 10,000 person-years

15. Assume that smoke and air pollution exert independent effects on COPD in question 14, rendering this joint effect multiplicative. Calculate the joint effects of these two variables in the multiplicative model.

a. 1,000 per 10,000
b. 50 per 10,000
c. 2,000 per 10,000
d. 32,000 per 10,000
e. 16,000 per 10,000

16. In a case-control study relating smoking to cancer of the cervix in women, the investigators found the crude odds ratio to be 6.6 and the Mantel–Haenszel odds ratio, adjusted for age, to be 6.3. In addition, their stratified analysis by age indicated the following odds ratio by the three age groups for smokers relative to nonsmokers: (1) age 20–29 years, OR = 27.9; (2) age 30–39 years, OR = 5.9; and (3) age 40+, OR = 2.8. Based on these results, age is considered to be a:

a. Positive confounder
b. Negative confounder
c. Nuisance covariate
d. Effect measure modifier
e. Confounder

17. Methods for controlling for confounding at the analysis phase of a study include all of the following *except*:

a. Standardization
b. Randomization
c. Stratified analysis
d. Matched analysis
e. Multivariate analysis

18. The following statements are all advantages of prospective cohort study *except*:

a. Recall bias is minimized compared to case-control designs
b. It is relatively inexpensive compared to case-control design
c. Precise measurement of exposure is possible
d. Incidence rate can be estimated
e. A number of disease outcomes can be studied simultaneously

19. The accompanying table presents the age group, number of person-years, and the mortality rate in standard population.

Age Group	Number of Person-years	Mortality Rate in Standard Population per 100,000	Expected Number of Deaths
25–34	7,557	0.8	
35–44	4,023	4.8	
45–54	2,961	47.9	
55–64	2,043	265.8	

If the total observed mortality from lung cancer is 12, what is the standardized mortality ratio?

a. 7.10
b. 12.0
c. 0.59
d. 1.69
e. Cannot be estimated from the information on the table

20. Regarding a case-control design, all of the following statements are accurate, *except*:

a. Recall bias is a potential problem
b. There is a possibility of having multiple comparison group

c. Disease rates are compared for subjects with the factor of interest and for those without the factor of interest
d. The proportion of cases with exposure is compared with the proportion of controls with the exposure
e. The odds ratio is the measure of the association

21. Which of the following is *correct* regarding ecologic fallacy?

a. Occurs when assessing exposure in large groups rather than small groups
b. Occurs when assessing outcomes in large groups rather than in small groups
c. Occurs due to investigator's inability to assess temporal sequence in causal inference
d. Occurs when an investigator attributes the characteristics of a group to every individual in the group
e. None of the above

22. An observational study (case-control) was conducted to determine the association between male hormone (testosterone, dihydrotestosterone, sex hormone-bidding globulin, and androstenidione) and prostate cancer among 1,850 U.S. residents aged 45 years and older. The investigators observed dihydrotestosterone as a risk for prostate cancer with an odds ratio of 2.6. What are the possible explanations for this finding?

a. Causal association
b. Chance association
c. Spurious association
d. a and c only
e. All of the above

23. The mortality rate in population A differs from the mortality rate in population B based on the crude comparison. Epidemiologists often utilize age-adjusted rates. This rate is used to:

a. Assess the coefficient of determination of mortalities in the populations
b. Correct the death rates for errors in the statement of age
c. Determine the actual number of deaths that occur in specific age groups
d. Remove the effects of differences in the age distributions of populations in comparing death rates
e. Compare the relative risk of dying in the two populations

24. The prevalence of a disease is an indication of the status of a disease in the population and does not provide information on the cause of the disease. The incidence of the disease reflects the new cases of the disease in a population. There is relationship between the prevalence and the incidence of the disease as well as the duration. If the incidence rate of gout is 5 times greater in women than in men, but the prevalence proportion indicates no sex difference, which of the following statements is most accurate?

a. The case fatality rate for gout is greater for women
b. The crude all-cause mortality rate is greater for women
c. The case fatality rate for gout is lower for women
d. The duration of gout is shorter in men
e. The predisposing factor for gout is more common in women

25. In a case-control study of osteoporosis, investigators examined 100 women as case and an equal number of women as control, and found low calcium intake in 40 of the cases and 20 of the controls. What is the odds ratio in the association between low calcium intake and developing osteoporosis in this population?

a. 1.53
b. 15.3
c. 2.66
d. 26.6
e. Cannot be estimated from the information provided

26. In a trial of an antiretroviral drug for AIDS treatment, the investigators reported 4 deaths among 55 patients treated with this agent, compared with 14 deaths among 52 controls on placebo. Calculate the attributable benefit of this agent in reducing mortality associated with AIDS in this study population.

a. 19.6%
b. 1.96%
c. 7.3%
d. 26.9%
e. 1.93%

27. Clinical trial is considered a gold standard in terms of epidemiologic designs. The purpose of random assignment in clinical trial is to:

a. Minimize selection bias in the allocation of treatment
b. Enhance double blinding
c. Facilitate the measurement of the exposure variables
d. Facilitate the measurement of the outcome variable
e. Control for confounding (comparable baseline characteristics)

28. Double blind design is often used in clinical trials. The purpose of double masking or blinding in these studies is to:

a. Minimize sampling error
b. Minimize interviewer bias
c. Minimize confounding due to observation
d. Ensure comparability of treated (treatment) and untreated (control) subjects
e. Reduce the effects of surveillance bias

29. A case-control design selects subjects based on disease, whereas cohort design selects subjects on the basis of exposure. Which of the following is a case-control study?

a. A study of cancer in men who have quit smoking
b. A study of the incidence of osteoporosis in women with low calcium injection
c. Obtaining histories and other information from a group of known cases and a comparison group to determine the relative frequency of exposure under study
d. A study of proportionate mortality using cumulative cases
e. Analysis of previous research to establish a summary point estimate

30. Epidemiologic causal inference relies on some set of criteria, especially those of Bradford Hill and Richard Doll. Which of the following is inaccurate when making causal inference using Hill's criteria?

a. Positive predictive value
b. Strength of association
c. Dose-response relationship
d. Temporality
e. Specificity

31. Bias is a systematic error arising from inaccurate measurement. Compared with prospective cohort study, which of the following biases is *most commonly* associated with case-control design?

a. Interviewer bias
b. Surveillance bias
c. Recall bias
d. Lead time bias
e. Non-response bias

32. Which of the following statements are *correct* concerning confounding?

a. Distortion of an exposure-outcome association is due to the association of another factor with both outcome and exposure
b. To be a confounding, a factor has to be independently associated with both exposure and outcome under consideration
c. Both of the above
d. None of the above

33. Regarding recall bias:

a. It occurs when the level of accuracy differs between the compared groups
b. It occurs in case-control studies when cases remember or report information differently from control
c. It occurs in prospective cohort studies when individuals who are exposed remember/report subsequent illnesses differently than those who are unexposed
d. a and c only
e. All of the above

34. Sources of epidemiologic data include all the following, *except*:

a. Vital statistics
b. National Health and Nutrition Examination Survey
c. National Health Interview Survey
d. Behavioral risk factors surveillance systems
e. None of the above

35. Which of the following statements is *correct* concerning cross-sectional study?

a. Examines the rate of disease in relation to population-level factor
b. The units of analysis are population rather than individual
c. Defines subjects according to exposure level and follows them for disease occurrence
d. Defines cases of disease and controls and compares the exposure histories
e. Cannot infer the temporal sequence between the exposure and disease

36. In a country with a population of 3 million people, 30,000 deaths occurred during the year ending December 31, 2005. These included 15,000 deaths from malaria in 50,000 people who were sick with malaria. What was the case-fatality rate from malaria in 2005?

a. 0.3%
b. 30%
c. 33.3%
d. 1.0%
e. None of the above

37. A graduate student is expected to interpret the study on the association between breast cancer and a high-fat diet. In the process of preparing his/her defense for the interpretation, s/he wishes to reflect on chance variation (random error), observation bias (systematic error), and confounding (the mixing effect of an external factor on the association between a high-fat diet and breast cancer. Which of the following should s/he consider first in the interpretation of the study?

a. Confounding
b. Random error
c. Observation (measurement) bias
d. a and c simultaneously
e. None of the above

38. Which of the following measures expresses the degree to which risk for a specific outcome is due to a specific exposure?

a. Absolute risk
b. Absolute risk increase
c. Absolute risk reduction
d. Attributable risk percent
e. Attributable risk

39. Publication bias is one of the issues confronting the use of the interpretation from meta-analysis for decision-making regarding interventions. Which of the following statements is accurate regarding publication bias in the conduct of meta-analysis?

a. Publication bias exists if the results of a study influence whether it is published or presented, or whether it is easily retrieved
b. The most likely effect of publication bias is that small studies, which show strong, significant, or unusual results, are more likely to be published than small studies, which show null results, or results in the expected direction
c. Both of the above
d. Neither of the above

40. A fixed-effect meta-analysis was conducted to examine the overall survival benefit of long-term versus short-term androgen deprivation therapy (ADT). The authors reported a hazard ratio (HR) of 0.52, 95% CI = 0.39−0.68, and chi square (χ^2) for homogeneity test = 4.5, with 4 degrees of freedom, $p = 0.4$. Which of the following interpretations could be made from these data?

a. Compared with short-term ADT, long-term ADT significantly increased overall survival by 48%
b. Compared with short-term ADT, long-term ADT significantly increased overall survival by 52%

c. Compared with short-term ADT, long-term ADT non-significantly increased overall survival by 48%
d. Compared with short-term ADT, long-term ADT non-significantly increased overall survival by 52%
e. None of the above

ANNOTATED ANSWERS

1. The answer correct is **D** (meaning of epidemiology). Epidemiology refers to the study of the frequency, patterns, causes, and control and prevention of diseases, disabilities, and injuries in the human population. There are two main aspects of epidemiology: (a) distribution—epidemiology evaluates the distribution of health states by age, gender, race, geography, time, etc., and (b) epidemiology seeks to examine the association and causal association between the exposure and the health-related states or events (Last, J.M., *A Dictionary of Epidemiology*, 3rd ed., 1995; MacMahan, B, & Trichopoulos, D., *Epidemiology, Principles & Methods*, 2nd ed., 1996, p. 1).

2. The correct answer is **E** (factors influencing the prevalence of disease). Prevalence proportion does not measure disease onset but the disease status. Whereas incidence is a measure of risk, prevalence is not because it does not take into account the duration of disease. But prevalence is related to the duration of the disease and incidence of disease. Prevalence = Incidence × Disease duration. The number of people living with a disease (prevalence) will be influenced by the rate at which a new disease develops as well as the rate at which they are eliminated through cure (prognosis) or death (mortality). Therefore, the prevalence will increase if incidence increases and if there is improvement in treatment but not cure, and it will decrease if there is dramatic cure (quick recovery) (Gordis, L., *Epidemiology*, 3rd ed., 2004, p. 40; Aschengrau, A., & Seage, G.R., *Essentials of Epidemiology*, 2003, pp. 48–49).

3. The correct answer is **E** (descriptive epidemiology).

4. The correct answer is **B** (primary attack rate). Attack rate, which is really a proportion and not a rate, is useful for comparing the risk of disease in groups with different exposures. This measure is calculated by Number of people at risk in whom a certain illness develops/Total number of people at risk. Substituting, 35/80 × (multiplier) = 35/80 × 100 → 43.75 per 100 (Gordis, L., *Epidemiology*, 3rd ed., 2004, p. 25).

5. The correct answer is **A** (secondary attack rate). Secondary attack rate yields the index of the spread of a disease within a family, household, dormitory, dwelling unit, etc. This measure is estimated by Number of new cases in a group − Initial case(s) / Number of susceptible persons in a group − Initial case(s). Substituting: 150 − 100 (each household had one primary case and there were 100 households) /500 − 100 (primary case) × 100 → 50/400 × 100 = 12.5% (Mausner, J., & Kramer, S., *Epidemiology—An Introductory Text*, 2nd ed., 1985, pp. 280–281).

6. The correct answer is **B** (relative risk/risk ratio). This is the measure of the strength of relationship between exposure and disease. Mathematically, RR = Risk or rate in the exposed/Risk or rate in the unexposed. Substituting: (46/68) / (13/59) → 3.07, implying that those exposed to egg salad had 3 times the increased risk of developing group A streptococci (Aschengrau, A., Seage, G.R., *Essentials of Epidemiology*, 2003, pp. 67–68; Mausner, J., Kramer, S., *Epidemiology—An Introductory Text*, 2nd ed., 1985, p. 169).

7. The correct answer is **E** (study design). A design that begins with exposure(s) of interest and disease-free subjects and aimed to assess the outcome in the future by following the subjects represents a prospective cohort study. This is not a clinical trial or a broad intervention design because the subjects of the FHS were not assigned but observed. The time relation in a prospective cohort study is present and future (continuing). A case cross-over design uses the previous experience of the cases as a substitute for a control series

to estimate the person-time distribution in the source population. Ambidirectional cohort is a design that is both retrospective and prospective in its observation of the outcome. Retrospective cohort (historical cohort studies) is a design in which the cohorts are identified from recorded information and the time during which they are at risk for disease occurred before the beginning of the study. Simply, retrospective study is conducted by defining the cohort and collecting information, which applies to past time. Case control is a design in which the groups of individuals are defined in terms of whether they have or have not already experienced the outcome under consideration, and the exposure is then measured (Elwood, J.M., *Critical Appraisal of Epidemiological Studies in Clinical Trials*, 2nd ed., 2003, pp. 14–35; Rothman, K.J., *Epidemiology, An Introduction*, 2002, p. 89).

8. The correct answer is **E** (study design). This is an observational design because it involves natural observation without assignment. A case control is a design in which the outcome had already occurred prior to the commencement of the study, and study participants were selected on the basis of the disease. The direct measure of risk is not possible in case-control study but estimated as odds ratio.

9. The correct answer is **E** (observational versus experimental design). Experimental design if feasible is considered the gold standard compared with observational studies. The active manipulation or assignment of the treatment by the investigator is the hallmark that differentiates experimental designs from observational studies. Whereas not all experimental designs utilize blindness to minimize bias, blindness is not a feature of observational designs. Neither in observational design nor experimental ones are investigators required to manipulate the outcome. Experimental designs, like observational ones, are conducted in human as well as animal populations (Aschengrau, A., & Seage, G.R., *Essentials of Epidemiology*, 2003, pp. 163–165).

10. The correct answer is **E** (internal validity of study). Confounding is derived from Latin "*confondere*", meaning "to pour together," and it indicates the confusion of two supposedly causal variables so that part or all of the purported effect of one variable (exposure) is actually due to the other (confounder). Confounding variable is considered an extraneous variable because it competes with the independent variable in explaining the outcome. In a study conducted to assess whether exposure (*A*) causes disease (*B*), *C* is a confounding if (a) *C* (smoking) is associated with *A* (coffee drinking) in the population that produced the cases *B* (pancreatic cancer), (b) *C* (smoking) is an independent cause or predictor of *B* (pancreatic cancer), or (c) *C* (smoking) is not an intermediate step in the causal pathway between coffee drinking (*A*) and pancreatic cancer (*B*) (Hennekens, C.H., & Buring, J.E., *Epidemiology in Medicine*, 1987, pp. 287–293; Gordis, L., *Epidemiology*, 3rd ed., 2004, pp. 228–229).

11. The correct answer is **C** (study validity—bias). Because men with diabetes mellitus are more heavily monitored compared to men who are not, disease ascertainment may be better in the monitored population and may introduce surveillance bias (monitoring of one population [diseased] more than the other [disease-free]). This bias may lead to erroneous estimation of the effect of the disease in the monitored population, thus inflating the point estimate (RR, OR) (Gordis, L., *Epidemiology*, 3rd ed., 2004, p. 227).

12–13. The correct answers are **C** and **D**, respectively (study validity—confounding). In all subjects without stratification by BMI, there is a strong association between exercise and type II DM, with low exercise as a risk factor, RR = 4.2 (26.25/6.25), where 26.25 is the incidence in those with low exercise (105/4,000 × 1,000). The RR in those with BMI > 24.99 kg/m^2 = 3.0 (30/10) and that in BMI < 24.99 kg/m^2 = 3.0 (15/5). Regardless of BMI, the best estimate of the effect of exercise on type II DM is 3.0. The crude estimate of 4.2 is indicative of the confounding effect of BMI on the association between exercise and type II DM. Moreover, BMI itself is risk for type II DM, as comparison here shows that low exercise subjects are much more obese in terms of their distribution by person-years, 75% versus 25% (high exercise).

14. The correct answer is **A** (interaction). Assuming the additive model, the expected incidence rate for joint exposure to smoke and air pollution is 40 (baseline rate), which is the rate in those unexposed to either of the two exposures, + 360 (400 – 40), (which is the rate in those with smoke minus the baseline rate) + 160 (200 – 40), which is the rate in those exposed to air pollution minus the baseline rate. Substituting in the additive model: 40 + 360 + 160 = 560 per 10,000 person-years. Therefore, the incidence rate in those with joint exposure is 560 per 10,000 person-years.

15. The correct answer is **C** (interaction). Assuming the joint multiplicative effect of the two exposures, the relative risk for smoking is RR = 10(400/40), where 40 is the baseline rate, the reference (1.0), and the relative risk for air pollution is RR = 5 (200/40), again where 40 is the baseline risk. The joint relative risk is 50 (10 × 5). The expected incidence rate for the joint exposure is then computed by multiplying the joint relative risk by the baseline rate. Substituting: 40 (baseline rate) × 50 (joint relative risk) = 2,000 per 10,000 person-years.

16. The correct answer is **D** (effect measure modifier). Because the difference between the crude OR (6.6) and the M-H adjusted OR by age (6.3) is less than the difference considered to be significant in establishing confounding (10.0%), age is not a confounding or there is very little confounding by age. In addition, the odds of smoking in the different age groups are very different, indicative of the role of age as effect measure modifier. Statistically, the presence of differences in the stratified OR (stratum-specific OR) is indicative of the possibility of interaction (effect measure modifier). Age therefore modifies the effect of smoking on cancer of the cervix in women (Gordis, L., *Epidemiology*, 3rd ed., 2004, pp. 233–234; Aschengrau, A., & Seage, G.R., *Essentials of Epidemiology*, 2003, pp. 337–341).

17. The correct answer is **B** (study design). Randomization is one of the three main ways to control for confounding at the design phase of a study. This method, which is restricted to experimental design, ensures that the treatment assignment occurs in an unbiased manner and results in the balanced distribution of known and unknown confounders (Aschengrau, A., & Seage, G.R., *Essentials of Epidemiology*, 2003, p. 288).

18. The correct answer is **B** (case-control study). Case-control design is relatively inexpensive to conduct compared with prospective cohort design. In comparison to case control, this is one of the disadvantages of prospective cohort studies.

19. The correct answer is **D**. The standardized mortality ratio is calculated by the formula: Observed death/Expected death. To obtain the expected number of deaths, the number of person-years from each age group is multiplied by the age-specific mortality rate in the standard population. The observed number of deaths is then divided by the sum of expected number of deaths. Substituting, Observed (12)/Expected (7.10) = 1.69.

Age Group	Number of Person-years (*P*)	Mortality Rate in Standard Population per 100,000 (*R*)	Expected Number of Deaths (*R* × *P*)
25–34	7,557	0.8	0.06
35–44	4,023	4.8	0.19
45–54	2,961	47.9	1.42
55–64	2,043	265.8	5.43
Total			7.10

20. The correct answer is **C** (study design).

21. The correct answer is **D** (ecologic fallacy).

22. The correct answer is **E** (study validity). Epidemic study aims to establish the association between risk factors, often called exposure or independent variables, and the outcome/response variable, which could be a disease, disability, or injury. The presence of an association may be a result of a factual relationship between these variables, which is broadly termed causal. For association to be causal, both bias and confounding must be eliminated as possible explanations of the association. In contrast, association may be noncausal or artifactual, implying that the finding is either influenced by a bias or confounding (Aschengrau, A., & Seage, G.R., *Essentials of Epidemiology*, 2003, pp. 251–252).

23. The correct answer is **D** (rates comparison). The crude mortality rates are inadequate in comparing the mortality events of two populations because populations differ with respect to age distributions, with advanced age associated with increasing mortality. Therefore, to adequately compare two populations in terms of mortality rates, age-adjusted rate is preferable, which removes the confounding or differences imposed by the differences in the age distribution of the population (Friis, R.H., & Sellers, T.A., *Epidemiology for Public Health Practice*, 1996, pp. 91–92).

24. The correct answer is **A** (relationship between incidence, prevalence, and disease duration). The prevalence of disease (assuming low prevalence) is associated with both incidence and the duration of the disease. The prevalence is the product of the incidence and the disease duration ($P = ID$), where P is the prevalence, I is the incidence of the disease, and D is the disease duration. The duration of the disease is influenced by (a) fatality or mortality and (b) prognosis (recovery). If the incidence of the disease is higher in one population (A) than the other population (B) and the prevalence is the same in both populations, the possible explanations are (a) the case fatality for the disease is higher in population A, and (b) the recovery is quicker in population A (Aschengrau, A., & Seage, G.R., *Essentials of Epidemiology*, 2003, pp. 48–49).

25. The correct answer is **C** (measure of association in case-control study). The association between osteoporosis and low calcium intake in this design (case control) can be estimated with the odds ratio (measure of association in case control), which is the odds of exposure in the disease divided by the odds of the exposure in the nondisease. Using the 2×2 table, the odds ratio is mathematically given by AD/BC. Substituting, $(40 \times 80) / (60 \times 20) = 2.66$

(Garb, J.L., *Understanding Medical Research: A Practitioner's Guide*, 2000, pp. 33–35, 131–132).

26. The correct answer is **A** (measure of risk difference). The attributable benefit (same as attributable risk) is calculated by first calculating the mortality benefit in those exposed to the antiretroviral drug and the mortality benefit in those not exposed to the antiretroviral drug. The attributable benefit is the difference between the benefit in those exposed to the treatment minus the benefit of those in the unexposed. Substituting, (a) Mortality rate in the exposed = $4/55 \times 100 = 7.3\%$, and (b) Mortality rate in the unexposed = $14/52 \times 100 = 26.9\%$. The attributable benefit or risk is computed by mortality rate in the unexposed minus the mortality rate in the exposed. Substituting, $26.9\% - 7.3\% = 19.6\%$.

27. The correct answer is **E** (clinical trial).

28. The correct answer is **D** (clinical trial).

29. The correct answer is **C** (study design).

30. The correct answer is **A** (epidemiologic causal inference).

31. The correct answer is **C** (study validity bias).

32. The correct answer is **C** (criteria for confounding).

33. The correct answer is **E** (bias-systematic error).

34. The correct answer is **E** (sources of epidemiologic data).

35. The correct answer is **E** (study design).

36. The correct answer is **B** (measure of disease occurrence).

37. The correct answer is **C** (internal validity).

38. The correct answer is **D** (measures of risk). *Absolute risk* is the outcome of events divided by the population at risk. This measure identifies the actual events rate in the population in question. *Absolute risk increase* is the pre-intervention absolute risk plus the post-intervention absolute risk. This measure identifies the absolute increase in the rate of specific adverse events associated with an intervention. *Absolute risk reduction* is the pre-intervention absolute risk minus the post-intervention absolute risk. This measure identifies the absolute decrease in the rate of specific adverse events associated with the intervention. Attributable risk percent is the attributable risk divided by the risk in the exposed times 100. This measure expresses the degree to which risk for a specific outcome is due to a specific exposure. Attributable risk (AR) is computed by the risk in the exposed minus the risk in the unexposed, and provides the measure of absolute risk associated with the exposure.

39. The correct answer is **B** (publication bias in meta-analytic design).

40. The correct answer is **A** (hazard ratio interpretation).

Chapter 3

Principles and Methods of Biostatistics in Public Health

Larry Holmes, Jr.

OVERVIEW

Biostatistics is a tool for the epidemiologic assessment and monitoring of health status, needs, and risk factors in order for public health to fulfill its substance of disease control and health promotions. As a basic science of public health, *biostatistics* has been described as the development and application of statistical reasoning and methods in addressing, analyzing, and solving problems in public health; health care; and biomedical, clinical, and population-based research. Both descriptive and inferential statistics are essential components of applied statistics in public health research.

This chapter reviews the basic notion of statistics and the role of statistics in health, biological, and medical sciences. Distinction is made between descriptive statistics (measures and central tendencies and dispersions) and inferential statistics (hypothesis testing and conclusion from the sample). Vignettes are utilized to illustrate the application of the classic statistical notions to real-world situations. Several test statistics are presented with their assumptions and rationale in testing various hypotheses and addressing relevant research questions. The statistical techniques or methods are reviewed in detail (correlation analysis, linear regression, logistic regression, and Cox proportional hazards model). Logistic regression analysis is reviewed with examples, given its widespread use in public health. The critique of literature is presented with the intent to allow readers to grasp the practical importance of biostatistics in the appraisal of scientific literature.

I. Basic Notions of Statistics and Biostatistics

A. *Biostatistics/biometry*: statistics applied to biological sciences and health-related events.
   1. Making sense of health-related data.
   2. Making inference about a population of interest based on information obtained from a sample of measurements from that population remains the objective of applied statistics such as biostatistics.

B. *Statistics*: concerned with data (numbers that contain information) collection, management (organization), analysis, and interpretation.
   1. Statistics studies a sample of the population; thus, drawing inferences about a population is a major role of statistics in research.
   2. Statistics is used to objectify the conclusions made in observational and experimental studies in public health.

C. Statistical methods are used to:
   1. Measure and explain overall variation.
   2. Differentiate between random and meaningful variation.
   3. Facilitate the interpretation of data needed for risk factors understanding and intervention implementation.

D. Biostatistics, branch of applied statistics investigates and evaluates the nature of information gathered on biological, clinical, and health issues or conditions.
   1. The role of biostatistics in research commences from design of study through implementation and the manuscript preparation for results dissemination.

II. Population Characteristics

A. Statistics is about sampling, and sampling is used to estimate or approximate the "real" or "true" characteristics of the population under investigation or study.

B. *Sample* refers to cases, subjects, or study participants (smaller group or subset of population) who are selected from the larger group (population) to investigate the association between exposure and disease (e.g., to understand the association in the population, also termed source population in this illustration).
   1. *Vignette:* Consider a study to examine the association between blood pressure and oral contraceptives. If the investigator selects 200 undergraduate female students in a university with 5,000 female students, the sample represents the 200 female students. The result of the study will be used to draw inference on the entire population (5,000 female students).
C. *Scales* used to measure population characteristics include:
   1. *Continuous,* which refers to a measure that uses an infinite number of values [e.g., systolic blood pressure (millimeters), urine drug concentration, hematocrit (millimeters), height (centimeters), BMI (kg/m^2), etc.].
   2. *Discrete,* which refers to only a few possible values, and measured in categories or classes [e.g., sex (male/female), race, marital status, skin color].
   3. *Ordinal,* which refers to categorical measures with natural order (e.g., educational status, comorbidity index, and disease severity).
D. *Estimates* are the values of sample characteristics, so termed because they proximate the value in the larger population.
E. *Continuous* characteristics in a population are described with the mean and standard deviation (measure of how much individual values in the population vary from the mean)—appropriate descriptive statistics for continuous variables.
F. *Discrete* or categorical characteristics from a population are described with proportion or percentage and rate (special proportion with time as a denominator).
G. *Ordinal* characteristics in a population are described by using median (population midpoint of ordered data) or mode (most frequent value).

H. *Probability model* is used to infer the characteristics of the population from the sample inferential statistics, which attempts to answer the question as to whether the observed difference is a result of "chance."

I. *Accuracy* with respect to the sample estimate refers to how close the estimate is to the true value in the population from which the sample was obtained; it is the ability of measurement to be correct on average.

J. *Bias* is a systematic or differential error in an estimate, with the sources of bias including:
   1. Selection bias—occurring when the subjects selected for study are not representative of the source population, limiting generalization of the result.
   2. Misclassification/information bias, which may result from:
      a. Defect or inaccuracy in the measuring device.
      b. Inaccuracy in the observation or recording of the measurements.

K. *Precision* (degree of "chance" differential or random error), also termed reproducibility or reliability, refers to the variability in the estimate.

L. The ability of a measurement to give the same results or very similar results with repeated measurements of the same thing. For example, the greater the standard deviation (SD), the less precise an estimate the mean will be from the true population mean (μ).

M. The degree of precision or random error is measured by the size of its confidence interval (CI), that is, the range of values for which one is fairly confident/certain that the true value from the population lies.

N. CI can be computed using the standard error (SE), which is the function of variability in the sample.
   1. SE is measured by SD and the sample size (n). Mathematically, $SE = SD/\sqrt{n}$, where n is the sample size.

III. Descriptive Statistics

A. Making sense of data in public health research involves four basic steps: (1) data collection, (2) data summary, (3) data analysis, and (4) data interpretation/result presentation.

B. Summarizing data, organizing data, graphing, and describing numeric information are the functions of descriptive statistics.

C. Descriptive statistics is concerned with measures of central tendencies and measures of dispersion, as well as their graphic presentation.

D. A *parameter* is a measurement of a population that characterizes one of its features. An example of a parameter is the mode. The mode is the value in the population that occurs most frequently. Other examples of parameters are a population's mean (or average) and its variance.

E. Descriptive statistics refers to *parameters* [population value of a characteristic of a *distribution* (values of characteristics or variable along with the frequency of their occurrence)] used to describe the attributes of a set of data such as mean, standard deviation, proportion, and rate.

Table 3-1 Scales of Measurement/Types of Variables*

Type of Data	Description and Example	Sample Estimate Summary and Presentation
Nominal (qualitative)	Dichotomous, binary, categorical	Proportion, percentage displayed with bar chart, contingency table
Ordinal	Nominal scale with natural order; e.g., stage of tumors	Proportion and percentage, median, mode; displayed with bar chart, contingency table

Table 3-1 Scales of Measurement/Types of Variables* *(cont.)*

Type of Data	Description and Example	Sample Estimate Summary and Presentation
Numerical (quantitative)	Continuous or interval and discrete	Mean and standard deviation, median and mode; displayed with stem and leaf plot, histograms, box plots, frequency polygons, and percentage polygons

*The scale of measurement influences the summary and the display of information. Variable refers to any information that can vary.

F. *Vignette*: Consider a chemoprevention study to assess the protective effect of selenium in prostate cancer. To test this hypothesis, investigators collected data from 500 treatments and 500 controls. What should be the initial approach toward understanding these data at the end of the intervention?

G. *Solution*: Prior to analysis of these data, a bar graph could be used to show those in the control who developed prostate cancer relative to the treatment group at the end of the follow-up.

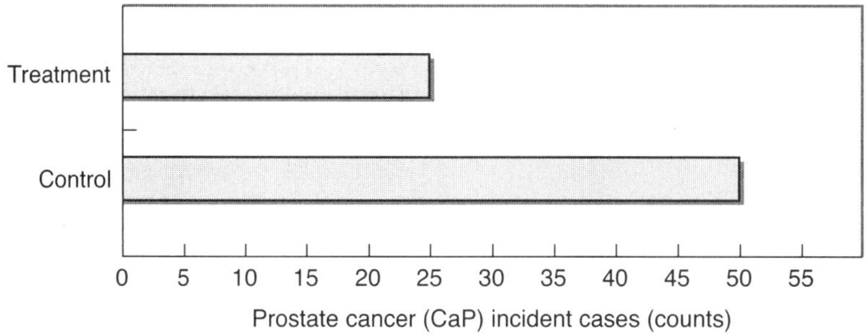

Figure 3-1 Incidence of Prostate Cancer among Healthy U.S. Male Adults in Selenium Chemoprevention Trial (Hypothetical Study)

1. *Measures of central tendency*
   a. The mean, median, and mode are the commonly used measures of location or central tendency.
   b. Whereas the *mean* (arithmetic mean) is the most commonly used measure of location, it is sensitive to extreme value (outliers) or skewed distribution, which makes it an inappropriate measure of central location in these types of samples.
   c. Mathematically, the mean is calculated by summing all the observations and dividing by the number of observation.
   d. Mean = $\Sigma X/n$, where Σ is the summation, X is the observation, and n is the number of observations.
      1. *Vignette*: Consider systolic blood pressure (SBP) of 10 women diagnosed with angina pectoris in a cardiovascular clinic ($x_1 = 102$, $x_2 = 144$, $x_3 = 110$, $x_4 = 138$, $x_5 = 130$, $x_6 = 120$, $x_7 = 140$, $x_8 = 100$, $x_9 = 60$, $x_{10} = 106$). What is the mean SBP in this sample?
      2. *Solution*: Mean (arithmetic) = Sum of the SBP/Number of SBP (subjects). Substituting: $(x_1 + x_2 + x_3 \ldots\ldots x_{10})/n$ → 115.
   e. *Median* is the middle value in an ordered or arranged data.
      1. It is an appropriate measure of central location when the data have outliers (skewed data).

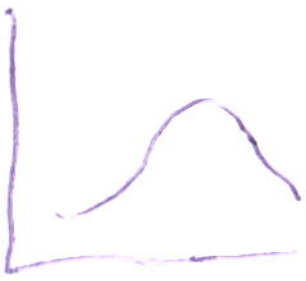

      2. *Skewed distribution* refers to outlying observations occurring in only one direction; thus, there are either a few small values or a few large values.

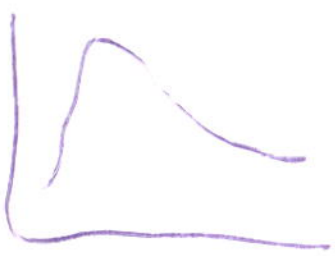

      3. *Positive skewness* occurs if the outlying values are large; thus, the distribution is skewed to the right.
      4. *Negative skewness* occurs if the outlying values are small; thus, the distribution is skewed to the left.
   f. *Mode* is the item with the highest frequency, or the value most frequently attained in a sample or population.
      1. Both the mode and median are not influenced by extreme high or low values or observations; thus,

they are useful in describing continuous variables/scale data whose values are not "normally" distributed.

Table 3-2 Uses of Measures of Location/Central Tendency*

Measures of Location	Statistical Utility
Mean	Numerical data
	Symmetric (nonskewed) data (distribution)
	Observations measured on a log scale (geometric mean)
Median	Ordinal data
	Numerical data with skewed distribution
Mode	Binomial distribution

*Suggestive of which measure of central tendency is best with a given set of data.

2. *Measures of dispersion*
   a. Measures of dispersion/spread are variance and standard deviation.
      1. Other measures of dispersion/variation are range, coefficient of variation, percentile rank, and interquartile range.
   b. *Range* is the difference between the largest and the smallest observations.
      1. *Vignette*: Consider the lowest mean arterial blood pressure (mmHg) of cocaine dependent patients in a drug rehabilitation clinic to be 108 and the highest to be 131. What is the range?
      2. *Solution*: The range is computed by subtracting the maximum from the minimum value. Substituting: 131 − 108 → 23 mmHg.
   c. *Coefficient of variation (CV)* is a useful measure of relative variation or spread in data.

d. CV is mathematically given by Standard deviation(*SD*)/ Mean(*X*) × 100 → *SD*/*X*(100), where *SD* is the standard deviation and *X* is the mean.
   1. This is a measure of relative variation, or the variation that is relative to the size of the mean.
e. CV is useful in laboratory testing and quality control procedures.
f. *Percentile* is the percentage of a distribution that is equal to or below a particular number.
   1. It is used to compare individual value such as height with the norm (e.g., a growth chart).
g. *Interquartile range* is the measure of variation that utilizes percentiles (e.g., the first and third quartiles are the 25th and 75th percentiles, respectively).
h. *Variance (square of SD)* is the standard dispersion of each observation from the group mean.
   1. Sum of squares/Sample size − 1($n - 1$), where $n - 1$ is the degree of freedom.
   2. $S^2 = \Sigma(X - M)^2 / n - 1$, where *M* is the mean of the sample, and S^2 is the biased estimate of $\sigma^2 = \Sigma(X - \mu)^2 / n$, where σ^2 is the variance in the population. But because samples are use to estimate the parameters, S^2 is the most commonly used variance.
i. Because the computation of variance involves the square of the dispersion of the observation from the mean, it does not provide a true measure of the average distance of each observation from the group mean.
j. *Standard deviation*: This is the square root of the variance → $\sqrt{\text{population variance}}$.
k. Mathematically: $\sigma = \sqrt{\Sigma(X - \mu)^2 / n}$
l. Square root of the average of the squared deviations of the observations from their mean is a more useful measure of dispersion for hypothesis testing.

Table 3-3 Steps to Calculate Variance and SD

- Calculate the mean, *X*.
- Prepare a table that subtracts the mean from each observed value $(X - M)$.
- Square each of the differences (different column) $(X - M)^2$.
- Add this column (sum of the squared dispersion from the mean) $\Sigma(X - M)^2$.
- Divide by $n - 1$ where n is the number of items in the sample (number of observations).
- This is the *variance*: $(S^2) \rightarrow (X - M)^2/n - 1$.
- To get the *standard deviation*, obtain the square root of the variance: $\sqrt{(X - M)^2 / n - 1}$.

1. Standard error simply stated as standard error of the mean is given by: $\sigma_m = \sigma / \sqrt{N}$, where σ_m is the standard deviation of the sampling distribution of the mean, σ is the standard deviation of the original distribution and *N* is the sample size (not assuming normal distribution).
2. *Standard error differs from Standard deviation*: (1) SE is the SD of a population of sample means, rather than of the individual observations, (2) refers to variability of the means, rather than variability of individual observations, and (3) provides idea of how variable a single estimate of the mean is likely to be.

Table 3-4 Uses of Measures of Dispersion

Measures of Dispersion	Statistical Utility
Standard deviation (SD)	Continuous data Mean Numerical data without skewness (symmetric numeric data)

Table 3-4 Uses of Measures of Dispersion *(continued)*

Measures of Dispersion	Statistical Utility
Percentile and interquartile range	With median (ordinal or skewed data)
	With mean (to compare individual observations with sets of numbers)
Interquartile range	To describe the central 50% of a distribution regardless of its shape
Range	With numerical data to stress extreme values
Coefficient of variation	To compare numerical distributions measured on different scales

IV. Types of Distribution

Table 3-5 Types of Distribution

Types of Distribution	Description and Example(s)
Normal (Gaussian)	Displayed as bell curve
	Data cluster around the middle or mean
	Fewer observations at either extreme
Parametric (also type of analysis, e.g., ANOVA)	Distributions that can be analyzed or estimated using parameters such as the mean and standard deviation, when the scale of measure or variable is continuous (e.g., *Z*-score, *t*-test, ANOVA)
Nonparametric (also type of analysis, e.g., chi-square)	Data that cannot be characterized by parameters such as mean and standard deviation
	Data that use nonparametric method such as chi-square

V. **Performance and Screening Test**

A. Screening is an effort to detect disease that is not readily apparent or risk factors for a disease in an at-risk segment of the population.

B. Diagnostic test, results, and implications of screening depend on both the prevalence of the disease and test performance.

C. Rare diseases are associated with relatively frequent false-positives relative to true-negatives.

D. Common diseases are associated with relatively frequent false-negatives relative to true-negatives.

E. Screening test is generally inappropriate when disease is either exceedingly rare or extremely common.

F. Measures of the diagnostic value of a test are its *sensitivity* and *specificity*.

Table 3-6 2 × 2 Table Comparing Test Results and Disease Status

Test Result	Disease Status: Diseased	Disease Status: Nondiseased	Total
Positive	*a* (diseased and positive)	*b* (disease-free and positive)	$a + b$ (all positive)
Negative	*c* (diseased and negative)	*d* (disease-free and negative)	$c + d$ (all negative)
Total	$a + c$ (all diseased)	$b + d$ (all nondiseased)	$a + b + c + d$

G. *Sensitivity* refers to the ability of a test to detect a disease when it is present.

1. Measures the proportion of those with disease who are correctly classified as diseased by the test.
2. Sensitivity = $a / a + c$ [Subjects with true-positive test results/(Subjects with true-positive results + Subjects with false-negative test result)].

3. A test that is not sensitive is likely to generate a false-negative result (c). False-negative error rate, Pr(T− | D+) = $c/(a + c)$, otherwise termed beta error rate or type II error.
4. Sensitivity [$a / (a + c)$] + False-negative error rate (FN rate), [$c / (a + c)$] = 1.0 (100%).

H. *Specificity* refers to the ability of test to indicate nondisease (disease-free) when no disease is present.
   1. Measures the proportion of those without disease who are correctly classified as disease-free by the test.
   2. Specificity = $d / (b + d)$ [Subjects with true-negative test results/(Subjects with true-negative result + Subjects with false-positive)].
   3. A test that is not specific is likely to generate false-positive results (b). False-positive error rate, Pr(T+|D-) = b / b + d(FP rate).
   4. Specificity ($d / b + d$) + FP rate [$b / (b + d)$] = 1.0 (100%).

I. *Predictive values* refer to: (1) the probability of having the disease being tested for if the test result is positive and (2) the probability of not having the diseases being tested for if the result is negative.

J. There are two types of predictive values used in diagnostic/ screening test:
   1. *Positive predictive value (PPV)*: The probability of a test being positive given that the disease is present.
   2. Mathematically: PD+ or PPV = a / {a + [(pT+ |D−)pD−)]} = a / {$a + b$}.

K. PD+ = True-positives / {True-positives + False-positives}. Using Bayes's theorem, PPV is the probability that an individual with a positive test result truly has disease, which is the proportion of all positives (true and false) that are true-positives.

L. PPV is thus the probability that a positive test result truly indicates the presence of disease.

M. *Sensitivity*: The probability of a positive test in those with the disease is the sensitivity ($a / a = c$).

N. *Prevalence*: The probability of the disease is the *prevalence* of the disease $(a + c) / (a + b + c + d)$.

O. Using Bayesian theorem: PD+ = (Sensitivity × Prevalence) / {[Sensitivity × Prevalence] + [(1 − Specificity)(1 − Prevalence)]}.

P. *Negative predictive value (NPV)* or PD: The probability of disease absence following a negative test result.

   1. NPV = True-negatives / {True negatives + False-negatives}→ $d / (d + b)$.

Q. *Using Bayesian theorem*: PD− = [Specificity × (1 − Prevalence)] / {[Specificity × (1 − Prevalence)] + [Prevalence × (1 − Sensitivity)]}.

R. *Likelihood ratios*:

   1. *Likelihood ratio positive (LR+)* refers to the ratio of the sensitivity of a test to the false positive error rate of the test.
      a. Mathematically: $LR+ = [a / (a + c) / [b / (b + d)]$.
      b. $LR+$ = Sensitivity / (1 − Specificity).
   2. *Likelihood ratio negative (LR−)* refers to the ratio of false-negative error rate to the specificity of the test.
      a. Mathematically: $LR- = \{c / (a + c)\} / \{d / (b + d)\}$.
      b. $LR-$ = (1 − Sensitivity) / Specificity.

S. Ratio of $LR+$ to $LR-$ refers to the measure of separation between the positive and negative test.

T. Mathematically, $LR+$ to $LR-$ ratio = $LR+ / LR-$. This is an approximation of the odds ratio. OR = ad / bc using 2 × 2 contingent table.

   1. *Odds ratio*: Odds of exposure in the disease/odds of exposure in the nondisease.
   2. *Odds of disease* (lung cancer) = Probability that lung cancer will occur (P)/Probability that it will not occur (1 − P).

U. *Vignettes*: Consider 160 persons appearing in a deep vein thrombosis (DVT) clinic for lower extremities Doppler ultrasound study. If 24 out of 40 subjects with DVT tested positive for DVT, and 114 out of 120 without DVT tested negative, calculate: (1) sensitivity, (2) specificity, (3) false-positive error rate, (4) false-negative error rate, (5) positive predictive value, (6) negative predictive value, (7) likelihood ratio positive, (8) likelihood ratio negative, (9) ratio of LR+ to LR−, and (10) the prevalence of DVT.

V. Generate a 2 × 2 contingent table.

Table 3-7 2 × 2 Table for DVT and Non-DVT

Test Result	Disease Status		
	DVT	**Non-DVT**	**Total**
Positive	24	6	30
Negative	16	114	130
Total	40	120	160

W. *Computation*: (1) Sensitivity = 24 / 40 = 0.6 (60%); (2) Specificity = 0.95 (95%); (3) FP error rate = b / (b + d) = 6 / 120 = 0.05 (5%); (4) FN error rate = c / (a + c) = 16 / 40 = 0.4 (40%); (5) PPV = 24(a) / 30(a + b) = 0.8 (80%); (6) NPV = 114(d) / 130(c + d) = 0.88 (88%); (7) LR+ = {a / (a + c)} = Sensitivity / {b / (b + b)} (false positive error rate) → 0.6 / 0.05 = 12.0; (8) LR− = False negative error rate {(c / (a + c) / Specificity {d / (d + b)} → 0.4 / 0.95 = 0.42; (9) LR+ to LR− ratio = LR+ / LR− = 12 / 0.42 = 28.57; and (10) Prevalence of DVT = (a + c) / (a + b + c + d) → 40 / 160 = 0.25 (25%).

X. Multiple or sequential testing refers to:
   1. *Parallel testing* (ordering tests together).
      a. The rationale is to increase sensitivity, but specificity is compromised.
      b. There are four possible outcomes in parallel testing: (1) T1+ T2+ (disease is present), (2) T1+ T2− (further testing), (3) T1− T2+ (further testing), and (4) T1− T2− (disease is absent).

1. *Sensitivity (net)* = (Sensitivity T1 + Sensitivity T2) − Sensitivity T1 × Sensitivity T2.
2. *Specificity (net)* = Specificity T1 × Specificity T2.
3. Individual tested positive on either test is classified as positive.
4. Appropriate when false-negative is main concern.

2. *Serial testing* refers to using two tests in series, with test 2 performed only on those individuals who are positive on test 1.
   a. There are four possible outcomes in parallel testing: (1) T1+ T2+ (disease is present), (2) T1+ T2− (negative), (3) T1− T2+ (negative), and (4) T1− T2− (disease is absent).
      1. Individuals must be positive in both tests to be classified as positive.
      2. Increases specificity but compromises sensitivity.
      3. *Sensitivity (net)* = Sensitivity T1 × Sensitivity T2.
      4. *Specificity (net)* = (Specificity T1 + Specificity T2) − Specificity T1 × Specificity T2.
      5. Appropriate when false-positive causes significant loss of subjects, and is of concern.

VI. Types of Variables, Random Variables, and Probability Distributions

A. *Variable* refers to a characteristic of interest in a study that has different values for different subjects.
   1. It is the measure of a single characteristic.

B. Sources of variation: (1) disease status, (2) biologic differences, (3) measurement conditions, (4) measurement methods, (5) measurement error, and (6) random error.
   1. Statistical methods/tools are used to make sense of the variation in data.

C. Types of variables in public health research:
   1. *Nominal variables* (naming or categorical) that have no measurement scales (e.g., skin color).

2. *Binary or dichotomous variable* or observation is a nominal measure that has two outcomes [e.g., gender (male → 1, female → 2), survival (yes → 1, no → 0)].
3. *Discrete variables* are binary and nominal, so termed because the categories are separate from each other [e.g., gender (male versus female)].
4. Ordinal variables are those with underlying order to their values [e.g., fatigue scale (0–10), absent, mild, moderate, severe].
5. Continuous or dimensional variables are characteristics that are measured on a continuum (e.g., systolic blood pressure, diastolic blood pressure, height, weight, age, etc.). Compared to ordinal, nominal, or discrete data, they allow for more detailed inferences.

D. *Random variable* refers to a variable in a study in which subjects are randomly selected. For example, if the subjects in a study to examine the survival of men treated for localized prostate cancer with radical prostatectomy are a random sample selected from the larger population, then race and Gleason score are examples of random variables.

E. *Probability distribution* is used to summarize values of random variable as a form of frequency distribution.

F. Types of probability distribution:
1. *Binomial* (yes and no) is a discrete probability distribution in which the associated random variable takes only integer values, 0, 1, 2, ..., n. It provides the probability that a specified event or outcome occurs in a given number of independent trials.
2. *Poisson* is a discrete distribution applicable, like binomials, when the outcome is the number of times an event occurs.
3. *Normal (Gaussian) distribution (bell-shaped curve)* is a continuous probability distribution. This distribution takes any value; it is a smooth, bell-shaped curve; and it is symmetric about the mean of the distribution, symbolized by μ, and a standard deviation symbolized by σ.

4. *Standard normal (Z) distribution* refers to the distribution with a mean of 0 and a standard deviation of 1. Mathematically, Z (Z-score, normal deviate, standard score or critical ratio) = $(X - \mu) / \sigma$.

VII. Sampling, Sample Size, and Power

A. Statistics deals with samples, and the main reason for research is to infer, or generalize, from a sample (sets of observations from one group of subjects) to a larger population (others who are similar to the subjects in the sample).

B. Statistics is the procedure by which some members of a given population are selected as representatives of the entire population.

C. The process of inference requires statistical methods based on probability.

D. Probability of a given outcome is the number of times that outcome occurs divided by the total number of trials.

E. Uses of probability: (1) understanding and interpreting data; (2) Indicating how much confidence there is in estimates such as the means, or relative risks; (3) understanding the meaning of p values.

F. *Probability rules:*

1. *Mutually exclusive events and the additional rule*: Two or more events are mutually exclusive if the occurrence of one precludes the occurrence of the others. The probability is found by adding the probabilities of two events (addition rule) → P(A or B) = P(A) + P(B).
2. *Independent events and multiplication rule*: Two events are independent if the outcome of one event has no effect on the outcome of the second (multiplication rule) → P(A and B) = P(A) × P(B).

G. *Population versus sample*: Population describes a large set or collection of items with common characteristics, whereas sample refers to the subset of the population, selected so as to be representative of the larger population.

H. *Why sample? "Bigger is not always better"*: (1) samples are quick to study; (2) they are less expensive; (3) it is difficult or impossible to study the entire population; (4) accuracy of result can be compared with the total population; (5) if properly selected, probability methods can be used to estimate the error in the resulting statistics, making a probability statement about the observations in the study; and (6) samples can be selected to reduce heterogeneity.
I. *Sampling techniques*: (1) probability sampling—ensures that a sample will lead to reliable and valid inference and (2) nonprobability sampling (unknown probability of selection)—deprived of the randomness needed to estimate sampling errors.
J. *Types of probability sampling*: (1) simple random sampling—in which every subject has an equal probability of being selected for the study; (2) systematic sampling—in which every *k*th item is selected, where *k* is determined by number of items in the sampling frame divided by desired sample size; (3) stratified sampling—in which the population is first divided into relevant strata or subgroups, and random sample is then selected from each stratum or subgroup; and (4) cluster sampling—in which the population is divided into clusters and a subset of the clusters is randomly selected.
K. *Sampling unit (element)*: Subject under observation on which information is collected (e.g., women aged 55 or older undergoing mammography).
L. *Sampling fraction*: Ratio between sample size and population size [e.g., 100 out of 4,000 (10%)].
M. *Sampling frame*: List of all sampling units from which sample is drawn (e.g., list of women aged 55 or older undergoing mammography).
N. *Sampling scheme*: Method of selecting sampling units from sampling frame (e.g., random selection, convenience sample).

O. *Sample size estimation and power*

1. *Sample size estimation*

   a. Sample size estimation for descriptive survey—one proportion. Using the formula for one proportion, $n = z^2 \times p \times q / d^2$, where n is the sample size, z is the alpha risk expressed in z-score, p = the expected prevalence and $q = 1 - p$, and d is the desired/absolute precision.

   b. Sample size estimation—two proportions or groups. Using the formula, $n = z_1 - \alpha/2[P_1(1 - P_1) + P_2(1 - P_2)] / d^2$, where n = sample size (each group), $z_1 - \alpha/2$ = confidence interval, P_1 = estimated proportion (larger), P_2 = estimated proportion (smaller), and d = desired precision.

2. *Statistical power*

   a. Probability that the test will reject a false null hypothesis.

   b. Probability that a study will not result in a type II error.

   c. The higher the power, the greater the chance of obtaining a statistically significant result when the null hypothesis is false.

   d. Depends on significance criterion as well as the effect size or the size of the difference.

VIII. Research Questions, Hypothesis Testing, and Statistical Inference (Testing)

A. Reading and interpreting scientific research requires understanding how research questions are formulated, hypotheses asserted, and specific test statistics selected to test the hypotheses.

B. Scientific finding, which commences with hypothesis testing and asserting an association, involves: (1) measurement of the magnitude of the outcome effect of interest by comparing outcome between groups with differing exposure; (2) measurement of variation among the observations of interest within exposure groups; (3) measurement of the ratio of outcome effect to variation (e.g., confounding); (4) elimination of alternative explanations (e.g., confounding, bias, random error-chance); and (5) ascertainment of association.

C. *Research question* refers to a statement that identifies the phenomenon to be investigated (e.g., "Does coffee drinking result in pancreatic neoplasm?").

D. Research questions could involve one group of subjects who are measured on one or two occasions. [For example, mean milk consumption and bone density in women 45 years and older. Appropriate research questions: (1) Is the mean milk consumption of women 45 years and older different in our sample compared with the National Study on Nutrition sample? In other words, how confident are we that the observed mean milk consumption in our sample is X oz/day? (2) Is the mean bone density (X) in the National Study on Nutrition of women 45 years and older significantly different from our sample?]

E. *What is the hypothesis*? To test or estimate the mean value of a numerical value (e.g., milk consumption, bone density). This hypothesis testing involves the examination of the mean in one group when the observations are normally distributed (e.g., bone density, milk consumption).

   1. *Test Statistic: t-test*

      a. *What is the test statistic?* The *t*-distribution is appropriate in performing the test statistics and obtaining the confidence limits.

      b. Simply stated, the single- or one-sample *t*-test compares the mean of a single sample to a known population mean.

      c. The purpose of this test (t) or student's *t*-test is to answer research questions about means.

      d. The formula for *t*-test is (Statistic − Hypothesized value) / Estimated standard error of the statistic. Mathematically: $t = (X - \mu) / (SD/\sqrt{n}) = (X - \mu) / SE$, where X is the observed or sample mean, μ is the hypothesized mean value of the population (true mean in the population), and *SE* is the standard error of the mean (X).

e. Simply, Mean(x) − Constant(μ) / SD(x), where SD(x) is the sum$\{(x_i - \text{Mean}(x)\}^2 / (n - 1)$.

f. To find out whether the observed mean is real [i.e., the observed mean is different from the mean of the National Study of Nutrition (NSN), termed the norm or population mean] and not just a random occurrence, the following factors need to be considered: (1) the difference between the observed mean and the norm (NSN) or population mean, implying much larger or smaller—magnitude of the mean difference → greater difference; (2) the amount of variability among subjects, implying less variation—smaller standard deviation in the sample (i.e., homogeneous sample and relatively precise method of measurement); and (3) the number of subjects in the study, implying larger rather than smaller sample.

   1. *Vignette*: Consider a study conducted to compare the mean vitamin C intake among 8th-grade school children at New School, Texas, with the population mean (Texas Study of Nutrition, or TSN). If the investigator found a greater standard deviation (SD), what is the probable explanation?
   2. *Solution*: If the SD is greater in the sample studied (8th-grade children at New School), it is likely that (a) vitamin C intake varies widely from one child to another, or (b) a crude measure devise is used to ascertain the vitamin C intake (improper, imprecise, or crude measure).

g. *Assumptions*: (1) Normal distribution. (2) If normality is not assumed, observations should be more than 30 subjects; thus means become normally distributed above this number regardless of the distribution of original observations (central limit theorem). (3) Even with violation of normal distribution, a *t*-test could still be performed since it is robust for non-normal data, implying the drawing of a proper conclusion even when the assumptions are not met, including normality.

h. *Interpretation*: The null hypothesis assumes the equality of means; a significant result at significance level (< 0.05) is indicative of the significant difference between the sample mean (X) and the population mean (μ). A nonsignificant difference implies that the difference may be due to random error or chance, given the significance level ($p > 0.05$), it does not mean that the two means are equal. Simply, one cannot be confident about accepting the observed difference because this might be due to random occurrence.

2. Types of *t*-test
   a. *An independent samples t-test* compares the means of two samples, with the assumptions that (1) two groups being compared should be independent of each other; (2) the scores should be normally distributed; (3) dependent variable must be measured on an interval or ratio scale; and (4) the independent sample should have only two discrete levels.
   b. *A paired samples t-test (dependent t-test)* compares the means of two scores from related samples, with the assumptions that (1) both variables are at interval or ratio scales; (2) both are normally distributed; (3) both are measured with the same scale; and (4) if different scales are involved, the scores be converted to *z*-scores prior to *t*-test analysis.

Table 3-8 Comparison between Standard Normal Distribution (*z*-score) and *t*-Distribution

Test	Description
z-score	Symmetric with mean of 0 and SE = 1.0
	Narrower and lower in tails compared to *t*-distribution. Why? Smaller SE.
t-distribution	Symmetric with mean of 0 and SE > 1.0
	Degree of freedom (df) is $n - 1$.
	Wider and higher in tails compared to *z*. Why? Larger SD.

c. Difference between *t* and *z* is very small when $n > 30$ subjects.

d. As sample size increases, degree of freedom (df) increases, and the *t*-distribution becomes almost the same as *z*.

e. With $n > 30$, either of the two distributions can be used.

f. *Other statistic for mean differences*: Because using a *t*-test involves a normal distribution and $n > 30$, another statistic for evaluating mean differences when these assumptions are not met is the Wilcoxon sign rank test (Mann–Whitney test), which is adequate for paired design as well as one sample.

g. Hypothesis testing about the proportion is performed using the *Z*-distribution.

   1. The process involves a research question [e.g., "Is there a significant difference in the observed proportion (0.20) of children with moderate to high physical activity in a sample, compared with the population proportion of 0.40?"].

h. Comparing two independent proportions involve the use of a *z*-test.

i. Comparing frequencies of proportion in two groups can be achieved with the chi-square test of independence.

j. Like the *t*-test, it is *z*-approximation (approximate test).

k. It is based on a null hypothesis of no difference/relationship/association or dependency.

l. A nonparametric procedure:

1. Research questions: (a) Is there a difference in the proportion of older men treated for prostate problems who received hormonal therapy relative to those who did not receive hormonal therapy? (b) Is there an association or relationship between women with autoimmune disorder and race?
2. Hypothesis (test the equality of these two proportions): The null hypothesis for dependency is that there is no racial difference among women with autoimmune disorders or simply, women with autoimmune disorders do not differ by race.
3. Mathematically: $\chi^2 = (O - E)^2 / E$, where O is the observed frequency, E = the expected frequency → $\chi^2_{(df)} = \Sigma$(Observed frequency − Expected frequency) / Expected frequency.
4. If no relationship exists, the observed frequencies will be very close to the expected frequency, thus rendering the chi-squared value small.
5. If more than 20% of expected, not the observed frequency, is < 5 → Fisher's exact test.
6. Assumption (same as one sample *t*-test): (a) The expected frequency for each category should be at least 1. (2) No more than 20% of the categories should have expected frequencies of < 5.
7. Test statistic: chi-square test of independence.
8. Interpretation: A significant chi-square test implies that two variables are not independent, meaning

that there is an association between the two variables, whereas a nonsignificant result indicates that the variables do not vary significantly from independence.

m. *Vignette*: Consider a study conducted to assess the relationship between gender and cardiomyopathies among U.S. residents. If the investigators found that men were 68% with cardiomyopathies while women were 40%, and the significance level was < 0.05, with a $\chi^2 = 27.32$, and df = 1, will you consider this finding to indicate that men are significantly more like to have cardiomyopathies relative to women?

   1. *Solution*: With the chi-square value (27.32), which is large, given 1 degree of freedom (3.84 critical value), and the p value, < 0.05, there is a significant association between gender and cardiomyopathies, leading to the rejection of the null hypothesis of independence or no association. Therefore, the conclusion drawn is accurate: men are more likely to have cardiomyopathies compared with women, based on the proportion in the result of the investigation.

n. Comparison of means in three or more groups involves the use of analysis of variance (ANOVA)—univariate or one-way ANOVA.

   Assumptions: (1) group independence (if subjects belong to more than one group → repeated measures ANOVA); (2) one independent variable (if more than one independent variable → factorial ANOVA (two-way ANOVA); (3) dependent variable is at interval or ratio levels, and is *normally distributed* → *parametric procedure*; (4) population variance is the same in each group (homogeneity of variance); and (5) observations are a random sample.

1. The test statistic for ANOVA (*F*-test) is not influenced by moderate departure from the assumption of normality, especially with large number of observations—*robust*.
2. Extremely skewed observations → Kruskal–Wallis test (nonparametric procedure).
3. Serious violation of ANOVA assumptions, as in t-test assumptions violation → Wilcoxon rank sum test (nonparametric procedure) for one-way ANOVA and Friedman test for one-way repeated measures ANOVA and two-way ANOVA (nonparametric procedure).

o. *Statistic*: *F*-test for two variances: ratio of the variance among means to the variance among subjects within each group.

p. *Hypothesis*: The null hypothesis is that the two variances are equal (i.e., the variation among means is not much greater than the variation among individual observations within any given group).

q. *Interpretation*: The *F*-value, degrees of freedom, and the significance level are necessary for the conclusion to be drawn on the significant mean differences between the groups.

r. Comparison of means in three or more groups with a covariate that is confounding involves the use of covariates (ANCOVA).

s. ANCOVA serves as a method of controlling for confounding.

IX. Analysis Techniques for Epidemiologic Data

A. Various test statistics are available for analyzing the relationship between two or more variables.

B. The selection of a test or statistic [e.g., *t*-test (testing for statistical significance)] depends on (1) the scale of the measurement of the dependent and independent variables, parametric (continuous scale data), or nonparametric (nominal/discrete scale data) distribution;

(2) the type of design (before and after comparison); and (3) the sampling procedure (random sampling), among other factors.

C. *Bivariate* or univariable analysis refers to the analysis of the relationship between *one* independent (X) and *one* dependent variable (Y). For example, if an investigator decides to examine the relationship between height and weight of 100 high school children, s/he may wish to determine if weight (Y) depends on height (X).

D. *Multivariable analysis* refers to the analysis between a single dependent variable and more than one independent variable (e.g., a study to determine the impact of race and gender in the development of colorectal cancer. The independent variables are age (X_1) and race (X_2), while the dependent variable is colorectal cancer (Y).

E. *Multivariate analysis* is the technique that involves more than one dependent and more than a single independent variable. This term is *not* interchangeable with multivariable analysis, and it is often used incorrectly.

Table 3-9 Analysis of Research Questions about Relationships among Variables: Correlation

Statistical Method	Variable	Assumption	Statistic
Correlation: Pearson	Dependent (outcome, response) and independent (predictors, explanatory) must be measured in continuous scale	1. Random sample 2. Bivariate normal distribution	Pearson product moment correlation coefficient (*r*)
Correlation: Spearman's rho/ Kendall tau	1. Numerical variables that are not normally distributed 2. Ordinal variables	1. Rank order data 2. Ordinal data, or interval or ratio 3. Nonparametric data	Spearman's rho or rank correlation (*r*)

F. *Correlation analysis*
   1. If either of the two variables is not normally distributed, Pearson correlation is considered inappropriate.
      a. *Alternate approach to analysis*: (1) Either one or both variables should be transformed to achieve near normal distribution. (2) Spearman rank correlation, which is a nonparametric test, should be used.
   2. *Interpretation*: (1) Correlation coefficient, r, is between -1.0 and $+1.0$, with r close to 0.0 considered to be a weak relationship. (2) 1.0 or -1.0 = strong relationship. (3) > 0.7 = strong correlation. (4) 0.3 to 0.7 = moderate correlation. (5) < 0.3 = weak correlation.

G. *Linear regression (least square regression) analysis*
   1. Refers to a regression method that is based on the least squares method:
      a. Linear regression is an analytic technique used to predict the value of one characteristic or variable (Y) from knowledge of the other (X). The regression equation is given by $Y = \beta_0 + \beta_1 X + \epsilon$.
      b. It is termed linear because this method, unlike correlation, measures only a straight line or linear relationship between two variables (simple linear regression).
      c. The least squares method minimizes the differences between the actual value of Y and the predicted value of Y $\{\Sigma(Y - \acute{Y})^2\}$, which is measured by the error term ϵ $(Y - \acute{Y})$ in the regression equation (G1a).
   2. In *simple linear regression* only a single independent or explanatory variable (X) is used to predict the outcome (Y).
   3. *Multiple linear regression* refers to a regression technique that, like the simple linear regression, is based on the

least squares method, where more than one independent variable is included in the prediction equation.

a. *Mathematically*: $Y = \beta_0 + \beta_1 X_1 + \beta_2 X_2 .... \beta_i X_i$, with β_0 and $\beta_{1...}\beta_i$ as the regression parameters.

4. Interpretation: The *simple linear regression* equation is given by $Y = \beta_0 + \beta_1 X + \epsilon$, where β_1 is the slope or the regression coefficient, β_0 is the intercept of the regression line (β_1 and β_0 are the population parameters), and ϵ is the error term, which is the distance the actual value of Y depart from the regression line.
5. *R square* (R^2) in the linear regression model output is the coefficient of determination that measures the proportion of the variance of the dependent variable (Y) that can be explained by the variation in the independent variable (X).
6. *The standard error of estimate* (model output) measures the dispersion for the prediction equation.
7. *Test statistics*: (1) ANOVA in the model uses *F*-statistic to determine the statistical significance of the regression equation and (2) *t* statistic test, whether or not the regression coefficient is statistically significant.

Table 3-10 Analysis of Research Questions about Relationships among Variables: Linear Regression

Statistical Method*	Variable	Assumption	Statistic
Simple linear regression (SLR)	1. Response is measured in continuous scale 2. Independent may be in continuous or binary scale	1. Both variables are interval or ratio scaled 2. Dependent (*Y*) must be normally distributed along the predicted line (homogeneity) 3. Relationship is linear	Regression statistic: (1) *t*-statistic (2) *F*-statistic

Table 3-10 Analysis of Research Questions about Relationships among Variables: Linear Regression *(continued)*

Statistical Method*	Variable	Assumption	Statistic
Multiple linear regression	Same as SLR; more than single dependent variables	Same as SLR; variables are also related to each other linearly	Same as SLR

*Performs the statistical test to determine the likelihood of any observed relationship between *X* and *Y* variables.

H. *Other types of regression (multiple)*
   1. *Polynomial regression,* which refers to multiple regression in which each term in the equation is a power of *X*.
   2. *Discriminant analysis* (predicts group membership with only two groups and uses continuous independent variables only) and *log-linear analysis* [focuses on the analysis of the conditional relationship of two or more categorical values; unlike binomial logistic regression, the dependent variable is categorical and the link function is the log (log of the dependent variable), not logit, and the predictions are estimates of the cells counts in contingency table, not the logit of the dependent variable, *y*].

I. *Logistic regression (LR) (binomial or ordinary)*
   1. Logistic regression is a form of regression analysis (logit transformation) where the outcome is binary and the independent variables could be measured in mixed scales (categorical, binary, mixed continuous and categorical).
   2. Logit transformation (logit p) for the binary outcome or dependent variable is denoted by: $\ln[p / (1 - p)]$, where the logit transformation takes any value from minus infinity to plus infinity.

3. This method calculates the probability or success over the probability of failure, thus presenting the odds ratio as the final result [e.g., logistic regression (LR) is used in determining the probability of developing prostate cancer, given exposure to organophosphates (pesticides) after adjusting for other known and postulated risk factors].
   a. Classified under generalized linear model (GLM).
   b. Also, the dependent variable can have more than two levels (e.g., multinomial and polytomous logistic regression).
4. Like SLR or MLR, logistic regression is a predictive model and is used to predict the outcome or dependent variable on the basis of continuous and/or binary/categorical independent or predictor/explanatory variables, as well as to determine the percent variance of the dependent variable that is explained by the independents, rank the relative importance of independents, assess the interaction effects, and control for confounding in the multivariable model.
5. This method uses maximum likelihood estimation after transforming the dependent variable into a logit variable, implying obtaining the natural log of the odds of the outcome or dependent variable occurring or not occurring—the probability of the outcome occurring.
6. The goal of this method is to correctly predict the outcome of the individual cases using the most parsimonious model.
7. Unlike the SLR, the relationship between the predictor and the response variables is not a linear function, but a logit transformation of the outcome variable.
8. The changes in the log odds of the outcome are estimated and not the changes in the dependent or outcome variable itself.
9. *Mathematically:* $\theta = e^{(\alpha + \beta_1 X_1 + \beta_2 X_2 + \ldots + \beta_i X_i)} / 1 + e^{(\alpha + \beta_1 X_1 + \beta_2 X_2 + \ldots + \beta_i X_i)}$, where α is the constant of the equation and β is

the coefficient of the predictor or independent variables in the model.

10. Given the probability of success (p) of a binomial outcome variable (y), the logistic regression model is: Logit (p) = $\ln(p / 1 - p)$ = alpha + $\text{beta}_1\ x_1$ + $\text{beta}_2 X_2$ + ... + $\text{beta}_k X_k$.
11. Likewise, solving for $p = e^{(\alpha + \beta_1 X_1 + \beta_2 X_2 + ... + \beta_k X_k)} / 1 + e^{(\alpha + \beta_1 X_1 + \beta_2 X_2 + ... + \beta_k X_k)}$.
12. The occurrence of outcome in this model is an exponential function of the independent variables: $Px = 1 / \{1 + \exp[-(b_0 + b_1 x_1 + b_2 x_2 + b_3 x_3 + b_4 x_4 + ... + b_i x_i)]\}$, where b_0 is the intercept (constant), b_1, b_2, b_3, b_4,..., b_i are the regression coefficient, while exp represents the base of the natural logarithm (2.718).
13. *Mathematically*, the odds ratio in LR can be computed from the coefficient of regression $\beta \rightarrow OR = e^{\beta}$, where exp = 2.718.
14. The Wald statistic (test) tests the statistical significance of the individual independent variable [each coefficient (β)] in the model.
15. The Wald test is a squared z-test with chi-square distribution: $Z = \beta / SE$ [coefficient (β)/standard error (SE)]. This is the squared ratio of the unstandardized logit coefficient to its standard error.
16. *Wald statistic interpretation*: Some statisticians have suggested that large logit increases standard errors, lowering the Wald statistic, thus leading to a type II error implying a false-negative, assuming that the effect is not significant, which indeed it is (rejecting the alternate hypothesis of difference).
17. *Model testing (appropriateness of the model)*: Goodness-of-fit (*Hosmer–Lemeshow*), which is a chi-square statistic with a desirable outcome of nonsignificance, indicates that the model prediction does not significantly differ from the observed.
18. *Model testing (backward stepwise elimination)*: Likelihood-ratio test (LRT) uses the ratio of the maximized value of the likelihood function of the full model (L_1) over the maximized value of the

likelihood function for the simpler model such as the model without predictors and or interaction (L_0). *Mathematically*: $\text{LRT} = -2\log(L_0 / L_1) = -2\{\log(L_0) - \log(L_1)\} = -2(L_0 - L_1)$.

19. The reduced model could be a baseline model or initial model with constant only, thus termed a null model. The full model then becomes the model with the predictors.
    a. A likelihood ratio test can then test the difference between the initial or null model, model with constant only, and the model with the coefficients from the predictors.
    b. The model is significant at $P < 0.05$, indicating that fitted model is significantly different from the null model or model chi-square test, as it is termed.
    c. This model does not ensure that every independent variable in the model is significant.
    d. Best model—the final model, which implies that adding another variable would not improve the model significantly (e.g., model with and without interaction).

Table 3-11 Analysis of Research Questions about Relationships among Variables: Logistic Regression

Statistical Method*	Variable	Assumption	Statistic
Logistic regression: unconditional (ULR)	*Outcome* is binary *Independent* variables are categorical and categorical and continuous (mixed)	Does not assume linear relationship Outcome need not be normally distributed Outcome need not be homoscedeastic for level of predictors No normally distributed error term	Wald statistic (β) Hosmer–Lemeshow (χ^2) (goodness of fit) Likelihood ratio test (overall model)

Table 3-11 Analysis of Research Questions about Relationships among Variables: Logistic Regression *(continued)*

Statistical Method*	Variable	Assumption	Statistic
Logistic regression: conditional	Same as ULR; matched pairs (1 − *K*)*	Same as ULR	Same as ULR

*Matching tends to increase the degrees of freedom relative to the cases. A better approach to the analysis is conditional logistic regression, which maximizes the likelihood estimate in logistic regression.

20. *Interpretation of logistic regression result* ($OR = e^{\beta}$): The odds in favor of success for a subject (*A*) (exposure = 1) is given by $OR_A = P_A / (1 - P_A)$, and the odds in favor of success for a subject (*B*) (exposure = 0) is given by $OR_B = P_B / (1 - P_B)$. The odds ratio is then $(OR) = OR_A / OR_B$.
21. The odds ratio relates a disease or outcome to the *i*th exposure for two hypothetical subjects *A* and *B*, where *A* is exposed and *B* is not.
    a. In the multivariable model, this odds ratio relates disease to the *i*th exposure variable, controlling for the levels of all other exposure variables in the model.

J. *Types of generalized linear models (counts data)*: Poisson regression, negative binomial regression, and zero-inflated regression models are appropriate for the analysis of count data which are: (1) highly non-normally distributed and (2) not well estimated by ordinary least squares (OSL) regression.

Table 3-12 Statistical Methods Involving Counts Data

Poisson regression	To model the number of occurrences of an event of interest or the rate of occurrence of an event of interest, as a function of some independent variables
	Efficient when the dependent variable is a count variable—with same length of observation time (e.g., number of days absent from work)
	Incidence rate ratio is the point estimate
Negative binomial regression	Used to estimate count models when the Poisson model is inappropriate due to over-dispersion (which is most of the time)
	In Poisson distribution the mean and variance are equal; thus, when the variance is greater than the mean, the distribution is said to display over-dispersion or lower than the mean, under-dispersion
	When there is over-dispersion, the Poisson estimates are inefficient with standard errors biased downward, yielding spuriously large *z*-values
	Efficient for dispersed count data, as an extension of generalized Poisson regression
Zero-inflated Poisson (ZIP) regression model	Extension of generalized Poisson regression with count data having extra zeros
	ZIP is useful to analyze such data
	Efficient where over-dispersion is assumed to be caused by an excessive number of zeros

K. *Statistical analysis method for event data (survival analysis)*

1. This method involves *censored observations* or data, where subjects have been observed unequal lengths of time and the outcome is not yet known for all subjects: left-censored if the episodes started before the period of observation and right-censored if the episode ended after the period of observation.

   a. Assesses the effect of independent variables on the event (what terminates an episode such as death in a clinical trial of drug or other therapeutics) in question.
   b. Simply, survival analysis assesses the simultaneous effect of several variables (covariates) on length of survival.
2. Time to event analysis or duration modeling is (1) parametric, where the shape of the baseline hazard function is assumed (e.g., *Weilbull model*), or (2) semi-parametric, where there is no assumption of the baseline hazard function shape but focus is on predicting the hazards ratio (e.g., Cox regression or proportional hazards model).
3. *Proportional hazard model (Cox regression)* refers to the hazard ratio remaining constant over time, which does not mean the *same* over time as often misinterpreted.
   a. This is Cox regression assumption: violation that may either overestimate or underestimate the point estimate (hazard ratio).
4. *Hazard, hazard rates, and ratios*
   a. *Hazard* is the event of interest occurring (e.g., death or biochemical failure in a clinical trial of a therapeutic agent).
   b. *Hazard rate* at a given time is the probability of the event given that the dependent = 1, occurring in that time period, given survival through all prior time intervals.
   c. *Hazard ratio,* also termed hazard function, refers to the estimate of the ratio of the hazard rate in group *A* (treatment group) to the hazard rate in group *B* (placebo group).
5. The survival function [$S(t)$] is the cumulative frequency of the proportion of the sample not experiencing the event by time *t* (alive or surviving observations).
   a. *Mathematically*: $S(t) = 1 - F(t)$, which is the probability that the event will not occur until time *t*, which also implies the proportion of participants surviving beyond any given time *t*.

6. The *survival function plot* enables the comparison of the survival rates of two or more groups in a study.
7. *Statistic*: (a) Likelihood ratio test for the model (sometimes *score statistic* is used); (b) regression coefficients (β) for the statistical significance of individual independent variables or covariates in the model; and (c) log-rank test for the equality of survival function.
8. *Interpretation*: Hazard ratio (HR), sometimes termed odds ratio, is given by exponent (β). If HR = 1.0, this means that the covariate (e.g., androgen deprivation therapy, or ADT in the model) has no effect or influence on the on time to event for the status or dependent variable (e.g., death from prostate cancer). If HR > 1.0, this indicates that the increases in the odds of dying given the use of ADT. Inversely, if HR < 1.0, this means that ADT diminishes or decreases the odds of dying on the subjects placed on ADT relative to those who are not.
9. *Survival curves estimation*: Kaplan–Meier survival analysis, also termed product-limit method, refers to a nonparametric method of generating tables and plots or graphs of survival, failure, or hazards functions for time to event data. (a) The assumption of the method is that the event must be dependent on time. (b) It involves the plotting of survival function on linear scale. (c) It is not designed to assess the effect or influence of covariates on the time to event status variable.

X. Critique of Scientific Literature—Interpreting Statistics in Public Health Research

A. Study designs: Determine the study design to address the research questions: (1) experimental (clinical trial, therapeutic, parallel, preventive, community, individual, etc.) and (2) observational (ecologic, cross-sectional, case-control, cohort, etc.).

B. Scale of measurement
   1. Determine the scale of measurement of the variables (nominal, categorical, discrete, ratio, interval) for the dependent and independent variables.
   2. Determine if data presented are assumed to follow normal distribution or not, parametric or nonparametric.
   3. If data are assumed to be normally distributed, are the descriptive statistics appropriate (mean, standard deviation, standard error, etc.)?
   4. If data are assumed to be nonparametric, are the descriptive statistics presented in terms of proportions, percentages?
C. Internal validity (random error, bias, and confounding).
D. Role of random error: Assuming a random sample was taken from the population studied, is this sample representative of the population? Is the observed result influenced by sampling variability?
E. The null hypothesis states that there is no association between the exposure and the disease variables, which in most instances translates to the statement that the measure of association = 1.0 (null), with the alternate hypothesis stated to contradict the null (one-tail or two-tail)—that the measure of association is not equal to 1.0.
F. *Significance level (alpha)*: The test statistics that depend on the design as well as the measure of the outcome and independent variables yield a p value. The p value (significance level) is the probability of obtaining the observed result and more extreme results by chance alone, given that the null hypothesis is true. The significance level arbitrary cutoff is at 5% (0.05). A $p < 0.05$ is considered statistically significant, implying that the null hypothesis of no association should be rejected in favor of the alternate hypothesis. Simply, this is indicative of the fact that random error is an unlikely explanation of the observed result or

point estimate (statistically significant). With $p > 0.05$, the null hypothesis should not be rejected, which implies that the observed result may be explained by random error or sampling variability (statistically nonsignificant).

1. *Vignette*: Consider a study to examine the association between physical inactivity and BMI among school-age children. Assume that the investigators found the risk of obesity (BMI > 30 kg/m^2) was 4 times higher among children with low levels of physical activity, and the p associated with the relative risk is 0.03. What is the possible explanation of this result, and is this result statistically significant?
2. *Solution*: (1) This simply means that if the null hypothesis is true, there is a 3% probability of obtaining the observed result or one or more extreme (RR = 4.0 or greater) by chance alone. (2) Because the p is < 0.05, the observed result is statistically significant.

G. *Type I or alpha error* refers to incorrect rejection of the null hypothesis, implying the rejection of the null hypothesis when indeed the null hypothesis is true.

1. When the null hypothesis is true and the investigator rejects the null hypothesis, type I error is committed (false-positive).

H. *Type II* or *beta error* refers to erroneously failing to reject the null hypothesis when indeed it is false.

1. When the investigator fails to reject the null hypothesis when it is false, type II error is committed (false-negative).

I. *Confidence interval (CI)*

1. Quantification of precision or random error around the point estimate, with the width of CI determined by random error arising from measurement error or imprecise measurement and sampling variability, and some cutoff value (95%).
2. CI simply implies that if a study were repeated 100 times and 100 point estimates and 100 confidence intervals were esti-

mated, 95 out of 100 confidence intervals will contain the true point estimate (measure of association).

3. CI is use to determine statistical significance of an association. If the 95% fails to include 1.0 (null), then the association is considered to be statically significant.
4. *Vignette*: Consider a study conducted to examine the role of passive smoking on lung carcinoma. If the 95% CI = 1.4 − 1.9, can we claim that there is a statistically significant association between passive smoking and lung carcinoma?
    a. *Solution*: Because the point estimate for the association lies within the upper and lower confidence limits, and 1.0 is not included, the observed result is statistically significant.

J. *Bias and sources of bias*
    1. Determine if bias, which is systematic error, contributes to the observed results.
    2. *Types of bias*: selection bias, prevalence or incidence bias (admission rate bias—Berkson's fallacy studying hospitalized patients as cases), nonresponse, and volunteer bias, etc.
    3. Measurement validity may introduce recall bias, detection bias, information bias, and compliance bias.

K. *Randomization and blinding (experimental and clinical trial)*
    1. Was randomization properly achieved?
    2. Was double blinding utilized?

L. *Power and sample size*
    1. Power measures the ability of the test to correctly reject the null hypothesis when the alternative hypothesis is true.
        a. *Mathematically:* Statistical power of a test = 1 − beta.
    2. Both alpha and beta errors are involved in sample size computation of a study.
    3. A small number is unlikely to show the difference between the two groups.

4. Sample size varies with the magnitude of the outcome effect expected. Thus, when variance is large, the outcome effect, even if robust, will be obscured by the underlying variation. Conversely, when the variation is modest, even modest effect may be perceived clearly with a small sample size.

REVIEW QUESTIONS (MULTIPLE CHOICE)

Directions: Each of the following questions contains multiple suggested responses. Select the *one best* response to each question.

1. The following table presents the STATA output of the mean baseline and 6 months' follow-up of systolic blood pressure of African-American men (n = 10), aged 35 to 48, treated with a daily beta blocker and a diuretic. Which of the following statement(s) is (are) *accurate*?

Paired *t*-Test

Variable	Obs	Mean	Std. Err.	Std. Dev.	[95% Conf.	Interval]
Baseline	10	124	3.42215	10.82179	116.2586	131.7414
Follow-up	10	112.6	2.62128	8.289217	106.6703	118.5297
Difference	10	11.4	1.681269	5.316641	7.596704	15.2033

Mean(diff) = Mean(Baseline − Follow-up)	$t = 6.7806$	
Ho: mean(diff) = 0	Degrees of freedom = 9	
Ha: Mean(diff) < 0	Ha: Mean(diff) != 0	Ha: Mean(diff) > 0
$Pr(T < t) = 1.0000$	$Pr(\|T\| > \|t\|) = 0.0001$	$Pr(T > t) = 0.0000$

a. The use of beta blocker and diuretic in these men with hypertension is associated with the decrease in the mean systolic blood pressure in this sample.
b. The paired *t*-test tests the null hypothesis that that the two population means are not equal.
c. The data assume that the paired scores of the subjects are normally distributed.
d. a and c only
e. None of the above

2. Understanding what *p* means requires understanding the logic of statistical hypothesis testing. For example, suppose an investigator wants to test whether or not Tamoxifen decreases breast cancer recurrence. He or she will select two groups of women diagnosed and treated for localized breast cancer through surgery and administer Tamoxifen to one group and placebo to the other. The odds ratio of breast cancer recurrence will be obtained comparing the two groups. To determine if the observed odds ratio is not due to random variation, an arbitrary cutoff point, termed a significance level, of 0.05 is often selected, and termed *p* value. Which of the following statements is *true* concerning the interpretation of the *p* value?

a. The probability of the sample data arising by chance
b. The probability of obtaining a value of the test statistic as large as or larger than the one computed from the data when in reality there is no difference between the different treatment groups
c. The probability of being wrong when asserting that a true difference exist between the two treatment groups
d. The chance of getting the observed effect if the null hypothesis was false
e. b and c only

3. An investigation was conducted to examine the relationship between serum cholesterol and BMI measured in kg/m^2. The study was analyzed using a correlation coefficient technique because the purpose of the design was not to use BMI to predict serum cholesterol level. Which of the following statement(s) is (are) *true* regarding this statistical method?

a. It only provides evidence of the causal relationship between two variables.
b. It is inappropriate when there is an underlying relationship between the two variables, but it is not linear.
c. It should only be used to judge the biological importance of the two variables.
d. It should not be performed unless the two variables are measured on continuous scale and are both normally distributed.
e. If the correlation is greater than zero (0), then serum cholesterol and BMI are said to be positively correlated.

4. A study was performed to determine neonatal weight (g) from maternal preconception weight (kg). A random sample of 100 mothers and their newborn babies (n = 100) were weighed. Which of the following statement(s) is (are) *accurate* regarding the interpretation or the statistical technique for the analysis of this study?

a. A two-sample *t*-test is adequate
b. Conditional logistic regression
c. Simple linear regression to describe the straight-line relationship between maternal preconception weight and neonatal weight
d. Neonatal weight (Y) can be predicted from maternal preconception weight (X)
e. c and d only

5. Most public health data involve the presence or absence of disease, termed binary outcome. The logistic regression model is an adequate predictive model in examining the association between an explanatory or independent

variable measured in continuous, categorical, or binary scale. Which of the following is (are) *correct* regarding the statistical model underlying the logistic regression model?

a. $\ln(P / 1 - P) = \beta_0 + \beta_1 X_1$
b. $Y = \beta_0 + \beta_1 X_1$
c. $\ln(P / 1 - P)$ = log odds (or logit) of disease risk
d. β_0 = log odds ratio associated with X_1 (exposure)
e. a and c only

6. The scale of variables is important in the selection of statistical methods. Which of the following statement/s is (are) *accurate* concerning dependent/response or outcome variable in linear and logistic?

a. Outcome is continuous in logistic model
b. Mean μ of outcome Y is $-\infty < \mu < +\infty$ in linear model
c. Outcome is categorical in linear model
d. P = Pr (disease) = logit (P) = $\ln(p / 1 - p)$ in logistic model
e. b and d only

7. African-American race/ethnicity is a known risk factor for hypertension. A study was conducted to determine the association between hypertension and salt intake in a sample of 250 white and 250 black males. The investigators utilized logistic regression model for their analysis in order to generate the coefficients (β) to relate hypertension to salt intake (X_1) and hypertension to race (X_2). What is the accurate interpretation of β_1?

a. Log odds of hypertension among the unexposed
b. Log odds of hypertension associated with salt intake
c. Change in the mean hypertension with a unit change in salt intake given that race is held at constant
d. Log odds of hypertension associated with race
e. None of the above

8. Low birth weight is an outcome that is a public health concern because infant mortality rates and birth defects are higher for low-birth-weight babies. Maternal behavior during gestation is a predisposing factor in pregnancy outcomes. As a public health statistician, if you are investigating the association between preconception obesity and low birth weight, and if there are age-matched controls (nonobese mothers), which of the following statistical techniques will be most adequate in the analysis of your data if the outcome (low birth weight) is binomial?

a. Unconditional logistic regression
b. Conditional logistic regression
c. Simple linear regression
d. Multiple linear regression
e. None of the above

9. A study was conducted to determine whether there is an association between daily exercise and colorectal cancer. The result indicated a relative risk of 0.8 and a 95% confidence interval, 0.7 – 1.3, for daily exercise relative to nondaily exercise in developing colorectal cancer over 10 years. The authors claimed that daily exercisers have a relative risk of 0.9 compared to nondaily exercisers in developing colorectal cancer over 10 years. Which of the following statements is *correct* regarding this finding?

a. The study had sufficient power to detect a true difference if one existed
b. The authors should have reported a 90% confidence interval
c. The authors are 95% confident that the null hypothesis is true
d. Type I error could have occurred
e. None of the above

10. A public health scientist wanted to calculate the linear association between low density lipoprotein (LDL) and prostate specific antigen. The two variables are continuous but the joint distribution is not Gaussian. Which of the following statistical methods may be *most* appropriate?

a. Simple linear regression
b. Spearman correlation coefficient
c. Pearson's correlation coefficient
d. Cox proportional hazards model
e. Poisson regression

11. A nutrition questionnaire was administered by e-mail to 837 U.S. male physicians on two separate occasions, 6 months apart. The questions to which responses were requested included the quantities of food eaten for 125 separate food items. The accompanying table displays the data obtained from the two surveys on the amount of fish consumed. Which of the following test statistics will produce the quantitative measure of reproducibility between the responses of the two surveys?

Amount of Fish Consumption Reported by 837 U.S. Male Physicians for Two Different Surveys

	Survey 1 ≤1 Serving/Day	**Survey 2 > 1 Serving/Day**	**Total**
≤1 serving/day	236	142	378
> 1 serving/day	119	340	459
Total	355	482	837

a. Chi-square statistic
b. Kappa statistic
c. Specificity
d. Spearman's correlation
e. Sensitivity

Questions 12–14 (*Fictitious Data*). Investigators conducted a study to evaluate the use of magnetic resonance imaging (MRI) in the diagnosis of brain attack. One hundred and sixty patients with brain attack confirmed by surgery were evaluated with MRI, as were 100 patients without brain attack. The MRI results were positive in 112 patients with brain attack and in 20 of the patients without the condition.

12. What is the false-positive rate in this study?

- a. 30%
- b. 20%
- c. 70%
- d. 80%
- e. 85%

13. What is the likelihood ratio positive of this test?

- a. 0.2
- b. 0.7
- c. 3.5
- d. 0.28
- e. None of the above

14. What are the chances of having a brain attack if the MRI is positive? Calculate the positive predictive value based on the given data in the table.

- a. 0.85 (85%)
- b. 0.15 (15%)
- c. 0.18 (18%)
- d. 0.70 (70%)
- e. None of the above

15. Which of the following statistical methods will be adequate to test the null hypothesis that maternal serum testosterone level, which is a postulated risk factor in testicular neoplasm, does not differ among African-American and Caucasian women, given that testosterone is measured in an interval scale and is normally distributed in these populations?

a. Mann–Whitney rank-sum test
b. Chi-square statistic
c. Unpaired *t*-test
d. Friedman statistic
e. Wilcoxon signed-rank test

16. In a study conducted to examine the correlation between alcohol consumption and systolic blood pressure in a sub-population of U.S. males, the investigators reported a significant positive correlation between these two variables. From this correlation, we may conclude that:

a. Subjects who consume less alcohol are at lower risk of increased systolic pressure
b. High alcohol consumption can cause increased systolic pressure
c. Subjects who consume less alcohol are at higher risk of increased systolic pressure
d. No association exists between alcohol consumption and systolic pressure
e. Low alcohol consumption can cause increased systolic pressure

17. Using statistical thinking to reach conclusions in epidemiologic and biomedical research amounts to much more than memorizing a few formulas and looking for *p* values in the tables. Applying statistical techniques and the results requires insights into the scientific hypothesis. All of the following should be clearly stated by the investigator regarding the scientific hypothesis, *except*:

- **a.** The name of the funding agency for the research and the affiliation of the principal investigator (PI) with the funding agency
- **b.** The data used to test the hypothesis
- **c.** The procedure used to collect the data
- **d.** The population the samples represent
- **e.** The statistical procedure used to evaluate the data and reach the conclusions

18. An epidemiologist wishes to study whether obesity is associated with prostate cancer. If, in reality, the presence of obesity leads to a prostate cancer relative risk of 3.0, the epidemiologist wants to have a 95% chance of detecting an effect this large in the planned study. This statement is an illustration specifying:

- **a.** Statistical power
- **b.** Odds ratio
- **c.** Hazards ratio
- **d.** Type I or alpha error
- **e.** Type II or beta error

19. A biostatistician observed a relationship between two measures (amount of contaminated water with fecal contents and frequency of diarrhea) to be linear and the coefficient of determination has a value near 1.0. A scatterplot of the observations will be:

- **a.** Horizontal straight line
- **b.** Vertical straight line
- **c.** Straight line that is neither horizontal nor vertical
- **d.** Random scatter of points about the regression line
- **e.** Positive slope

20. Holmes and colleagues (2007) conducted a study to determine the effectiveness of androgen deprivation therapy (ADT) on loco-regional prostate cancer. The authors reported that the effect of ADT on survival was assessed using Kaplan–Meier's method, a log-rank test, and Cox proportional hazards. Which of the following statement(s) is (are) true regarding the log-rank test in their analysis techniques?

a. Compares data on those who received ADT relative to those who did not
b. Tests the null hypothesis that each group (ADT and non-ADT) has the same force of mortality
c. Calculates the probability that the observed death would have occurred in the ADT group and the probability that it would have occurred in the non-ADT group
d. a and c only
e. All of the above

Questions 21 and 22. The accompanying table gives some of the results from the same study (Holmes et al., 2007). This table presents the multivariable result of the effect of ADT on the overall survival of older men treated for loco-regional prostate cancer.

Effect of Androgen Deprivation Therapy on Overall Survival of Older Men Treated for Local/Regional Prostate Cancer in 1992–1999 SEER Areas

Hazard Ratio (95% Confidence Interval) of All-Cause Mortality in Cases Receiving ADT, Primary Therapy, and Chemotherapy

	Model I		**Model II**	
Covariates	**HR**	**95% CI**	**HR**	**95% CI**
Androgen deprivation therapy (ADT)				
No	1.0	Reference	1.0	Reference
Yes	1.29	1.24–1.34	1.04	1.00–1.08

(continues)

Covariates	Model I HR	Model I 95% CI	Model II HR	Model II 95% CI
Primary therapy (PT)				
WW	1.0	Reference	1.0	Reference
RP	0.20	0.19–0.21	0.32	0.30–0.33
XRT	0.47	0.45–0.48	0.63	0.61–0.65
RP/XRT	0.29	0.26–0.32	0.40	0.36–0.45
Chemotherapy				
No	1.0	Reference	1.0	Reference
Yes	0.93	0.90–0.98	1.01	0.97–1.05

Notes: Model I adjusted for primary therapy and chemotherapy. Model II adjusted for sociodemographics, comorbidity, tumor characteristics, and primary therapies plus chemotherapy. Abbreviations: watchful waiting (WW) or observational management, radical prostatectomy (RP), radiation therapy (XRT), hazard ratio (HR), and confidence interval (CI).

Data from: Holmes, L., et al. Effectiveness of androgen deprivation therapy in prolonging survival of older men treated for loco-regional prostate cancer. *Prostate Cancer and Prostatic Diseases,* 2007, doi:10.1038/sj.pcan.4500973.

21. The hazard ratio for the effect of primary therapy (PT) on survival is presented with watchful waiting as the reference. What is the interpretation of the hazard ratio (HR) of 0.32 and a 95% confidence interval, 0.30–0.33, for the effect of radical prostatectomy (RP) on survival?

a. Surgery relative to watchful waiting or observational management significantly reduces the risk of dying by 68%

b. Surgery relative to watchful waiting or observational management significantly reduces the risk of dying by 32%

c. Watchful waiting relative surgery increases the risk of dying by 32%

d. There is a statistically nonsignificant 32% increased risk of dying in subjects undergoing watchful waiting compared with subjects undergoing surgery

e. There is a statistically nonsignificant 68% decreased risk of dying in subjects undergoing surgery compared with subjects undergoing observational management or watchful waiting

22. Based on the information in the table, what conclusion could be drawn from this study on the effect of ADT in prolonging survival of older men treated loco-regional prostate cancer?

- **a.** ADT significantly increases survival by 4%
- **b.** There was a nonsignificant decrease in survival due to the use of ADT
- **c.** ADT nonsignificantly decreased survival by 40%
- **d.** There was increased survival of 40% among the subjects who did not use ADT
- **e.** None of the above

23. Which of the following is (are) method(s) of depicting frequency distribution?

- **a.** Histograms
- **b.** Stem leaf
- **c.** Boxplots
- **d.** Quantiles
- **e.** All of the above

24. In an intervention program to control blood pressure among 36 inner-city African-American women aged 36 to 56 years, at the end of the intervention an investigator found the mean systolic blood pressure to be 123.1 mm Hg and a standard deviation of 11.3 mmHg. If a standard error (SE) is required to be calculated, what will this be?

- **a.** 1.88 mm Hg
- **b.** 2.02 mm Hg
- **c.** 10.89 mm Hg
- **d.** 3.42 mm Hg
- **e.** None of the above

25. A study examined glucose tolerance and insulin sensitivity in normal and overweight hyperthyroid-prone inner-city Hispanic-American women. If the authors wanted to compare the baseline glucose (mmo/L) in the women to see if weight or thyroid level have an effect, which of the following statistical methods would be *most* appropriate?

- **a.** Two-way ANOVA
- **b.** One-way ANOVA
- **c.** Logistic regression
- **d.** Paired *t*-test
- **e.** Correlation analysis

26. (Fictitious study) A study was designed to examine the relationship between children's age and daily consumption of apple and orange juices. There were 100 two-year-old children [$<$ 12 fluid ounces of juice/day (n) $=$ 75 and $\geq$ 12 fluid ounces/day (n) $=$ 25] and 85 five-year-old children [$<$ 12 fluid ounces of juice/day (n) $=$ 70 and $\geq$ 12 fluid ounces/day (n) $=$ 15]. The combined age (2 years and 5 years, $n = 185$) indicated that $<$ 12 fluid ounces of juice/day (n) $=$ 155 and $\geq$ 12 fluid ounces/day (n) $=$ 30. What is the *best* statistical method to determine whether or not there is difference between the 2-year-olds and 5-year-olds regarding the daily consumption of apple and orange juices?

- **a.** Pearson correlation
- **b.** Fisher's exact test
- **c.** Paired *t*-test
- **d.** Fisher's *z*-distribution
- **e.** ANOVA

27. Chlamydia trachomatis (CT) is an established pathogenic microbe in non-gonococcal urethritis, pelvic inflammatory disease, and other infectious diseases. An investigator wishes to conduct a study to examine the risk factors associated with CT using 862 female undergraduate students. He or she intends to control for several risk factors simultaneously in the analysis of variables associated with CT. If CT is measured in binary scale, which of the following analytic methods might be appropriate?

a. Multivariate logistic regression
b. Multivariable logistic regression
c. Simple linear regression
d. Stratified analysis
e. Conditional multivariable logistic regression

28. An investigator wishes to examine the relation between cholesterol as a risk for heart disease. If s/he chooses to measure cholesterol using an interval scale, which of the following scales will be adequate in measuring heart disease (outcome variable)?

a. Binary
b. Ordinal
c. Interval
d. Continuous
e. Quantitative

29. You are involved in a descriptive survey to examine the association between physical activities and overweight and obesity. If the sampling technique in the study involves simple random or systematic sampling, absolute or desired precision is 0.03, the prevalence of physical activity is 15%, and alpha risk expressed in *z*-score is 1.96, what will be an estimated sample size for this study?

a. 1,088
b. 544
c. 833
d. 163
e. None of the above

30. As a newly hired public health analyst, you are required to obtain a sample of 90 children from the Well Child Program for a study to assess the effect of vitamin supplements on childhood growth. There are 1,800 children in the sampling frame. All of the following will be accurate regarding your approach, *except*:

- **a.** The sampling fraction = 20
- **b.** Sampling frame list subjects from 1 to 1,800
- **c.** A number from 1 and 20 is randomly selected
- **d.** If the first person selected is 10th in the sampling frame, the second person will be the 32nd
- **e.** If the first person selected is 8th in the sampling frame, the second person to be selected is the 28th

ANNOTATED ANSWERS

1. The correct answer is **D** (assumption and interpretation of paired or dependent *t*-test). The paired *t*-test tests the null hypothesis of no difference or equality of the two means (baseline relative to follow-up). Because the difference is > 0, the use of these two anti-hypertensive agents is associated with a decrease in mean systolic blood pressure in this sample. Secondly, given the significance level, $p < 0.05$.

2. The correct answer is **E** (*p* value interpretation).

3. The correct answer is **E** (correlation coefficient).

4. The correct answer is **E** (simple linear regression).

5. The correct answer is **E** (logistic regression model).

6. The correct answer is **E** (characteristics of dependent variable in logistic and linear regression models).

7. The correct answer is **B** (interpretation of coefficient in logistic model).

8. The correct answer is **B** (analysis technique in matched-case control studies).

9. The correct answer is **D** (interpretation of 95% confidence interval).

10. The correct answer is **B** (nonparametric correlation regression).

11. The correct answer is **B** (reproducibility test). Reliability studies are designed to quantify the reproducibility of the same variable (e.g., daily dietary intake of a particular food), measured more than once. Kappa, which is a measure of agreement "beyond chance," is used as a measure of reproducibility between repeated assessments of the same variable. The chi-square test of association between the two surveys responses, although performable, will not give a quantitative measure of the reproducibility between the responses in the two surveys. Using kappa statistics (κ) is the appropriate test to measure reproducibility: $P_o - P_e / 1 - P_e$, where P_o is the observed probability of the concordance between two surveys, and P_e is the expected probability of concordance between the two surveys. kappa, $\kappa > 0.75$ (75%) indicates excellent reproducibility, 0.4 (40%) $\leq \kappa \leq$ 0.75 (75%) indicates good reproducibility, while $0 \leq \kappa < 0.4$ (40%) denotes marginal/poor reproducibility. In addition, +1.0 is indicative of a perfect agreement, while 0.0 indicates complete independence between the two surveys. Specificity and sensitivity would be more appropriate indices of reliability or reproducibility if the investigators were interested in the concordance between responses on two different variables, where one of the variables is considered to be the cold standard (Abrahamson, *Making Sense of Data*, 2nd ed., 1994, pp. 171–182).

12. The correct answer is **B** (diagnosis and screening test). False-positive error rate (alpha error rate or type I error rate) simply refers to an error committed by asserting that a proposition is *true*, when it is indeed *not true* (false). If a test is not *specific*, this will lead to the test falsely indicating the presence of a disease in nondisease subjects (cell B; see accompanying table). The rate at which this occurs is termed the false-positive error rate and is mathematically given by $B / (B + D)$. False-positive error rate is related to specificity: FP(rate) + Specificity = 1.0(100%).

Test Result	Brain Attack		Total
	Present	**Absent**	
Positive MRI	*A* (112)	*B* (20)	132
Negative MRI serving/day	*C* (48)	*D* (80)	128
Total	$A + C = (160)$	$B + D = (100)$	$(a + b + c + d) = 260$

Using the 2 × 2 contingent table, the false-positive error rate = $B / (B + D)$. Substituting: 20/100 = 0.2(20%).

13. The correct answer is **C** (likelihood ratio of screening test). The likelihood ratio positive illustrates the ratio of sensitivity of a test ($a / a + c$) to the false-positive error rate ($b / b + d$) of the test. Using the formula: $a / (a + c) / b\,(b + d)$; substituting: 0.7/0.2 = 3.5.

14. The correct answer is **A** (positive predictive value). The positive predictive value (PPV) answers the question, if the patient's test result is positive, what is the probability that he or she has the disease? PPV indicates the proportion of the subjects who had positive MRI, and had brain attack. Using the formula: PPV = $A / A + B$, substituting; 112 / (112 + 20) = 0.85 (85%).

15. The correct answer is **C**. An unpaired *t*-test is appropriate in testing the hypothesis comparing two groups that consist of different individuals when the measurement scale is interval and drawn from normally distributed populations.

16. The correct answer is **B** (interpretation of correlation analysis). Correlation analysis is conducted to determine whether or not there is a relationship or an association. A significant positive correlation suggests that the relationship is directly proportional, meaning that *Y* (response variable—systolic pressure) increases as *X* (independent variable—alcohol consumption) increases.

17. The correct answer is **A** (scientific hypothesis testing).

18. The correct answer is **A** (statistical power).

19. The correct answer is **C** (graphic presentation of data).

20. The correct answer is **E** (test of significance for differences in survival). Success or effectiveness of treatment is measured in terms of time that some desirable outcome is maintained. Such analysis (time-related patterns of survival) techniques originated from the life table procedures. Kaplan–Meier, also termed the product limit method, is more commonly used in biomedical and public health research compared to actuarial method. Kaplan–Meier product limit and actuarial methods are commonly used to estimate survival experience of samples. Both methods are similar except that time since entry in the study is not divided into intervals for analysis in Kaplan–Meier product limit method. Two or more life table curves could be tested to determine if they are significantly different. The *z*-test for proportion is used for the actuarial curves while the log-rank test is used for Kaplan–Meier curves. The log-rank test is an approximate chi-square test and compares the number of observed deaths in each group with the number of deaths that would be expected from the number of deaths in the combined groups, implying that group membership or distinction did not matter. The log-rank test is also referred to as the Cox–Mantel log-rank statistic or the Mantel log-rank statistic. The log-rank test, as may be incorrectly interpreted, does not involve ranking nor does it employ logarithm in its computation of the survival differences (Holmes,

Effectiveness of androgen deprivation therapy in prolonging survival of older men treated for loco-regional prostate cancer. *Prostate Cancer and Prostatic Diseases*, 2007, doi:10.1038/sj.pcan.4500973).

21. The correct answer is **A** (interpretation of hazard ratio in Cox proportional hazard model).

22. The correct answer is **E** (hazards ratio and 95% confidence interval interpretation).

23. The correct answer is **E** (methods used in illustrating frequency distribution).

24. The correct answer is **A** (calculation of the standard error). The standard error allows the investigator to estimate the probable amount of error of the quantitative assertions, as well as enables the performance of statistical significance test (95% confidence interval). The standard error is calculated using the formula $SE = SD/\sqrt{n}$, where n is the number of observations. Substituting: $11.3/6 = 1.88$ mm/Hg. Please note that the larger the sample size (*n*), the smaller the standard error and the better the estimate of the population mean will be. Because SE can be converted to SD and vice versa, SD and SE are both acceptable measures of the amount of errors around the quantitative assertions.

25. The correct answer is **A** (two-way analysis of variance).

26. The correct answer is **B** (Fisher's exact test). When one or more of the expected, not the observed, counts in a 2×2 table is small (< 2), the chi-square test cannot be used; instead, the exact probability of finding the observed numbers by using Fisher's exact probability test is employed.

27. The correct answer is **B** (analysis of binary outcome data with several independent variables on mixed scales, controlling simultaneously for other variables).

28. The correct answer is **A** (scale of measurement of variables).

29. The correct answer is **B** (sample size estimation for descriptive survey). Using the formula for one proportion: $n = z^2 \times p \times q / d^2$, where n is the sample size, z is the alpha risk expressed in z-score, p = the expected prevalence and $q = 1 - p$, and d = the absolute precision. Substituting, $1.96^2 \times 0.15 \times 0.85 / 0.03^2 = 544$.

30. The correct answer is **E** (systematic sampling).

Chapter 4

Behavioral and Social Sciences in Public Health

Larry Holmes, Jr., and Doriel D. Ward

OVERVIEW

Behavioral science, which embraces psychology, sociology, and anthropology, has been described as the study of actions and reactions of humans and other animals, using experimental and observational methodologies. The application of these disciplines to the health of the population represents its affiliation with public health. The behavioral and social sciences in pubic health address the behavioral, social, and cultural factors related to individual and population health and health disparities over the life cycle. Research and practice in this area contributes to the development, administration, and evaluation of programs and policies in public health and health services to promote and sustain healthy environments and healthy lives for individuals and populations. Therefore, behavioral science is a cross-fertilization between applied public health disciplines and management and policy sciences.

To maintain that there are rarely any health conditions without a behavioral input or influence is as true as maintaining that to every physical disease process, there is an emotional reaction. The role of behavior in risk and predisposing factors to acute and chronic diseases has been well illustrated, as well as the application of behavioral interventions in reducing disease risk factors, increasing compliance to intervention and treatment regimens, and improving disease prognosis and reducing mortality.

Whereas the specific mechanisms have not been fully understood, it is plausible that behavior intervention, involving knowledge of health-related events risk or predisposing factors, may enhance skills toward risk avoidance or compliance to treatment, and hence improve the overall health outcomes. The social determinants of health have been clearly demonstrated. Inequity in education, income, and socioeconomic status has been associated with variances in disease presentation, screening, treatment received, and health outcome (including mortality). This chapter reviews the basic concepts in behavioral sciences and their relations to health promotions; health theories and models (e.g., the theory of reasoned action), social and psychological determinants of health, and health disparities.

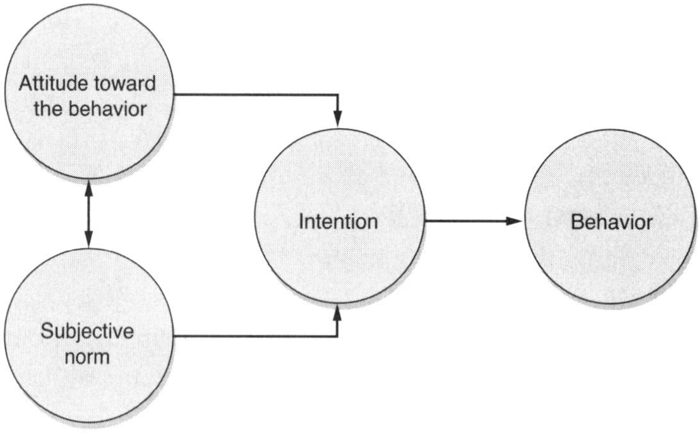

Figure 4-1 Theory of Reasoned Action

I. Notion of Behavioral Sciences and Its Role in Health Promotions and the Prevention of Health-Related Events

A. Health and disease are determined by dynamic interactions among biological, psychological, behavioral, and social factors or variables.
   1. These interactions occur over time and throughout the life cycle.

B. The health of the public is integrally linked to social, behavioral, physical, biologic, and economic environments.

C. Psychological factors influence health directly through biological mechanisms and indirectly through arrays of behaviors.

D. Social and psychological factors that influence health include: (1) socioeconomic status, (2) social inequalities, (3) social network and support, (4) work conditions, (5) depression, (6) anger, and (7) hostility.

E. *Behavior*, which is the collectivity of acts, is fundamental to health outcomes, health promotion, and disease prevention.

F. The Healthy People 2010 initiative demonstrates the potentials for change in behavior or behavior modification in reducing morbidity and mortality in most of the leading causes of death in the United States.

G. *Behavioral sciences* refers to a multidisciplinary (sociology, anthropology, psychology) approach to the study of actions and reactions of humans and other animals through observational and experimental methods.

H. The behavioral sciences dimension of public health involves the use of sociologic, anthropologic, and psychological methodologies in understanding health behaviors, and the application of this knowledge in designing interventions to promote health and prevent diseases, injuries, and disabilities (health-related events).

I. Whereas the substance of public health is disease prevention and health promotion, social sciences enhances health promotions by indicating:
   1. How people think about their behavior.
   2. How people determine their risk (risk perception).
   3. How people change their behavior.
   4. How people cope with health issues/problems.

J. *Behavior change*: Deciding to change behavior depends on:
   1. Beliefs about current health status:
      a. General health values.
      b. Risk perception.
      c. Vulnerability.
      d. Self-efficacy.
      e. Response efficacy.

2. Impression management, which implies the influence of one's health behavior from the social perspective of one's behavior.
3. Intentions versus willingness, with willingness as a better predictor of behavior change relative to the intention to change behavior.

Table 4-1 The Importance of Behavior in Health (Morbidity and Mortality), Healthy People 2010

- The major leading causes of death (heart disease, cancer, and stroke) in the United States are associated with behavioral (lifestyle) variables.
- Reduction in heart disease morbidity and mortality can be achieved through smoking cessation, cholesterol lowering (dietary regulation), and exercise (physical activities).
- Significant decline in cancer death (lung, renal) can be achieved through smoking cessation.
- Substantial reduction in stroke can be achieved by controlling hypertension, regular exercise, dietary regulation, and smoking cessation.
- Significant reduction in auto accident mortality can be achieved by eliminating drunk driving.

K. *Health determinants (illustrative)*: The key determinants of health include biologic, social, behavioral, and psychosocial variables or factors, which may be illustrated as follows:
1. *Hereditary*: Genetic predisposition plays an important role in obesity, most tumors, some chronic diseases, and emotional disorders such as schizophrenia. For example, prostate cancer tends to run in families, which is indicative of the possible role of gene, physical environment, or gene-environment interaction.
2. *Childhood development*: Chronic diseases such as childhood hypertension have been associated with early uterine and

early developmental effects. For example, the failure to thrive has consequences beyond childhood.

3. *Gender*: Gender predisposes to some behavioral risk factors and health conditions. For example, (1) men are more likely to be aggressive compared to women; studies using the Y chromosome explain this variation in aggressiveness. (2) Early-onset hypertension is more common in men than in women. (3) Autoimmune disorders such as systemic lupus erythematosus (SLE) are more common in women than men. Whereas no reliable explanation for the gender variation is available for SLE, it is plausible to suggest the role of estrogen, as well as screening bias, because men are less likely to seek medical care and as such are less likely to be diagnosed relative to women.
4. *Coping skills*: Teaching individuals more adaptive coping skills may help reduce risky behavior.
5. *Personal health practices*: For example, breast self-examination may help discover breast lumps or cysts and may help in the diagnosis of early-stage breast tumors.
6. *Social environment*: Interpersonal relationships in family and social network settings have been shown to improve health conditions.
7. *Physical environment*: Environmental exposure influences the likelihood of developing a disease. For example, (1) cancers and asthma have been linked to air pollutants (tobacco and asbestos) and (2) childhood neurologic deficit has been associated with exposure to lead-based paints.
8. *Employment status and working condition or environment*: Being unemployed is associated with impecunity, which influences access to health care, thus compromising screening and early diagnosis of treatable conditions (e.g., breast cancer, prostate cancer). Also, being employed and not having health insur-

ance through that employment may increase the risk of morbidity for the same reason—reduced access to care. Further, uncomfortable working conditions may lead to a predisposition to stress in the first place and subsequent clinical conditions associated with high stress (hypertension, angina pectoris, coronary artery disease).

9. *Educational status*: Higher educational status is associated with employment, high income level, access and utilization of health care (racial/ethnic majority), and knowledge of risk factors (all races/ethnicity), all of which are variables/factors associated with improved health outcomes.
10. *Social support network*: Improved health outcomes.
11. *Family support system*: Improved health outcomes.
12. *Income and social class status*: The most important determinant of health and disease prognosis and mortality is income, which translates to social class (higher, middle, and lower) not race/ethnicity.
13. *Cultural and racial/ethnic background*: Membership in a racial/ethnic group is associated with incidence, prevalence, and disease prognosis, as well as mortality. Race/ethnicity is a complex phenomenon and, like education, is associated with income, employability, access, and utilization of health care and knowledge of risk factors. African Americans, relative to Caucasians, bear the burden of disease disproportionately because this group is less educated and is therefore less likely to be employed; 80% live below poverty level, lack health insurance coverage, are less likely to receive early diagnosis, and hence have poor prognosis and increased mortality from most causes of death relative to their Caucasian counterparts.
14. *Age*: Chronologic (physical) age is associated with disease incidence, prevalence, and mortality. For example: (1) Children and elderly are more predisposed to infectious diseases because

of the compromization of the immune system. (2) Elderly are more vulnerable to chronic disabilities and chronic diseases. (3) Children are vulnerable to leukemia (nonsolid tumors), whereas advancing age is associated with most tumors (except germ cell testicular neoplasm, with the peak age of onset at age 29 to 34 years).

15. *Access to health services*: Early diagnosis and improved prognosis.
16. *Utilization and quality of health care*: Early diagnosis and improved prognosis.

L. *Health promotion* is the combination of educational, organizational, policy, financial, and environmental supports to reduce disease, disability, and injury risk factors and to promote healthy lifestyles.

M. Health promotion is achieved by:

1. Following an objective such as Healthy People 2010.
2. Identifying healthy people who are engaged in risky behaviors.
3. Assisting individuals in their pursuit of specific behavior change.
4. Motivating people to change their actions and reactions.
5. Providing intervention that increases the likelihood of success.

N. Behavior change is influenced by (1) predisposing factors, which are: (a) knowledge, (b) beliefs, (c) attitudes, (d) gender, (e) age, (f) race/ethnicity, and (g) socioeconomic status; (2) enabling factors, including (a) skills and abilities and (b) available resources; and (3) reinforcing factors, such as (a) family support system, (b) social support network, and (c) motivation, or wanting or willingness to change behavior.

O. Behavior change strategies: (1) shaping, (2) visualization, (3) modeling, (4) controlling the situation, (5) reinforcement, (6) self-talk changing (improving one's image to encourage the change in behavior), (7) self-assessment, (8) personal behavior analysis, (9) decision making, and (10) realistic goal setting.

II. Health Demographics and Health Disparities (Inequity)

A. *U.S. Demographics*

The U.S. Population by Race and Hispanic Origins, 2000 and Projected 2050, indicates that:

1. In 2000, non-Hispanic Whites totaled 274,595,678, more than two-thirds (75.1%) of the total population (n = 281,421,906).
2. By the year 2050, the U.S. Census Bureau predicts the proportion of the population that is non-Hispanic White will diminish to just over half the total population.
3. Black or African Americans totaled 34,658,190, less than one-fifth (12.3%) of the total population.
4. American Indians/Alaska Natives (AI/AN) totaled 2,475,956 (0.9%) of the total population.
5. African-American and American Indian/Alaska Native (AI/AN) populations are also expected to increase.
6. Asian Americans totaled 10,242,998 and Native Hawaiian/ Pacific Islanders (AAPI) totaled 398,835 (3.6% and 0.1%, respectively) of the total population.
7. The largest increase is expected in the Asian-American/Pacific Islander (AAPI) population, which is expected to almost triple its current size by 2050.
8. Hispanics or Latinos totaled 35,305,818 and non-Hispanics or Latinos totaled 246,116,088 (12.5% and 87.5%, respectively) of the total population.
9. The Hispanic/Latino population is expected to almost double by 2050.
10. Two or more races totaled 6,826,228, while some other race totaled 15,359,073 (2, 4, and 5.5%, respectively) of the total population.

B. *Racial Disparities in Health and the Measure of Disparities*

1. *Health disparities* refer to absolute and relative differences, disease rates, and health outcomes affecting the health status of certain race/ethnic, age, and gender groups, as well as socioeconomic/social class and geographic area/locale (e.g.,

Blacks and American Indians have diabetes at higher rates than Whites).

2. *Absolute and relative inequalities (racial/socioeconomic model)*
   a. The health gap between racial/socioeconomic groups can be considered in both relative and absolute terms.
   b. *Relative measure*: An example of a relative measure would be the ratio of the death rate in the lowest social class or one racial group (White) to that in the highest class/other racial groups (Black, Asian, Hispanic, or Latino).
   c. Death rates could be, for example, twice as high in Blacks as in Whites.
3. *Absolute measure* refers to the rate difference, which is computed by subtracting the death rate in one group from that in another *(rate difference)*.
   a. This could be expressed as, for example, the death rate in Blacks (rates in Blacks = 75 deaths per 100,000) is 50 deaths per 100,000 greater than the rate in Whites (rates in Whites = 25 deaths per 100,000).
   b. Both relative and absolute measures have important implications.
   c. Absolute measures are the most critical *(program planning and intervention)*, particularly with respect to identifying the major problems that need to be addressed. This is because an absolute measure is determined not only by how much more common the health problem is in one group than another, but also by how common the underlying problem (e.g., the death rate in a particular population) actually is.

C. *Racial and ethnic minority populations*
   1. Dramatic and persistent health disparities have been described among the following groups:
      a. American Indian/Alaska Native (AI/AN): People having origins in any of the original peoples of North and South America (including Central America), and who maintain tribal affiliation or community attachment.

   b. Asian American: People having origins in any of the original peoples of the Far East, Southeast Asia, or the Indian subcontinent.
   c. Black or African American: People having origins in any of the black racial groups of Africa.
   d. Hispanic or Latino: A person of Cuban, Mexican, Puerto Rican, South or Central American, or other Spanish culture or origin, regardless of race.
   e. Native Hawaiian or Other Pacific Islander (NHOPI): People having origins in any of the original peoples of Hawaii, Guam, Samoa, or other Pacific Islands.
2. Disparities in health are observed in racial/ethnic background, with discrimination and bias of healthcare providers indicated as playing a fundamental role, illustrated as follows:
   a. Blacks are less likely than Whites to receive certain procedures and treatment (after controlling for income, education, and personal characteristics).
   b. Clinicians (doctors) in a study rated Blacks as less intelligent, less educated, more likely to use drugs and alcohol, less apt to comply with medical advice, and more likely to lack social support.
   c. Among Medicare recipients in managed care health plans, Blacks were less likely to receive (1) breast cancer screening, (2) eye exams when diabetic, (3) medicine after heart attack, (4) flu shots, and (e) follow-up care after hospitalization for mental illness.
   d. Asthmatic African Americans in one health maintenance organization (HMO) were less likely than Whites to see specialists and to use inhalers and were more likely to be hospitalized.
   e. Blacks with diabetes are less likely to get proper medical care than White diabetics.

D. *Racial disparities in major causes of death and other conditions for disparities elimination*

1. Age-adjusted mortality rates (U.S., 2002) per 100,000 persons by race/ethnicity for three health focus areas (heart disease, cancer, stroke):
   a. African Americans have the highest all-cause death rate (1,083.3 per 100,000), and the highest death rate for three of the leading causes of death. They also lead in deaths from diabetes (49.5 vs. 25.4 per 100,000 for all populations); homicide (21.0 vs. 6.1 per 100,000 for all populations); influenza and pneumonia (24.0 vs. 22.6 per 100,000 for all populations); and breast, prostate, and lung cancer (34.0, 62.0, and 61.9, respectively, vs. 25.6, 27.9, and 54.9, respectively, per 100,000 for all populations).
   b. African Americans have a higher cancer death rate than White Americans, even though White Americans have a higher prevalence of cancer: 7.8% for Whites, compared to 3.4% for African Americans, which is suggestive of some racial disparity in cancer screening and/or treatment.
   c. African-American, American Indian, and Puerto Rican infants have higher death rates than White infants. In 2000, the Black-to-White ratio in infant mortality was 2.5 (up from 2.4 in 1998). This widening disparity between Black and White infants is a trend that has persisted over the past two decades.
   d. African-American women are more than twice as likely to die of cervical cancer as are White women and are more likely to die of breast cancer than are women of any other racial or ethnic group.
   e. Heart disease and stroke are the leading causes of death for all racial and ethnic groups in the United States. In 2000, rates of death from diseases of the heart were 29%

higher among African-American adults than among White adults, and death rates from stroke were 40% higher.

f. In 2000, American Indians and Alaska Natives were 2.6 times more likely to have diagnosed diabetes compared with non-Hispanic Whites, African Americans were 2.0 times more likely, and Hispanics were 1.9 times more likely.

g. Although African Americans and Hispanics represented only 26% of the U.S. population in 2001, they accounted for 66% of adult AIDS cases and 82% of pediatric AIDS cases reported in the first half of that year.

h. In 2001, Hispanics and African Americans aged 65 and older were less likely than non-Hispanic Whites to report having received influenza and pneumococcal vaccines.

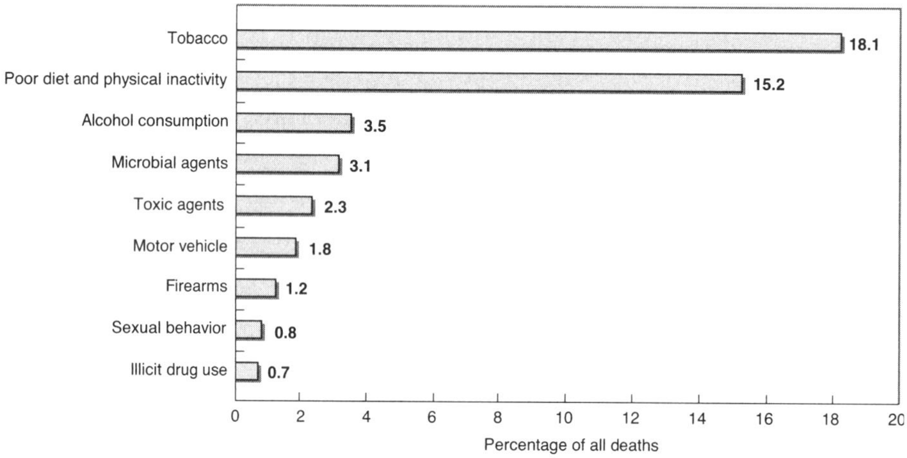

Figure 4-2 Leading Predisposing Factors of Death (Actual Causes) in the United States, 2002

Source: Mokdad, Marks, Stroup, & Gerberding. Actual causes of death in the United States, 2000. *JAMA*, 291: 1238–1245 (2004).

E. *Other health disparities measures*
   1. Health disparities have been described among other populations, namely:
      a. Socioeconomic status.
      b. Geography (urban or rural).
      c. Gender.
      d. Age.
      e. Disability status.
      f. High-risk status related to sex and gender.

F. *Sources of disparities in health:*
   1. Ethnicity and race (income, poverty).
   2. Racial/ethnic discrimination (clinician's bias and prejudice).
   3. Lack of and limited insurance coverage (income).
   4. Lack of access to transportation and other barriers to access to health services (income).
   5. Health services utilization (income).
   6. Access and utilization of quality care (income).
   7. Lifestyle variables.
   8. Cultural variations.
   9. Dietary patterns (income and lifestyle).
   10. Lack of exercise.
   11. Obesity and overweight.
   12. Inadequate maternal and child health (poverty).
   13. Environmental factors (income, which determines where individuals reside).
   14. Stress and mental health (income and utilization of preventive health services).

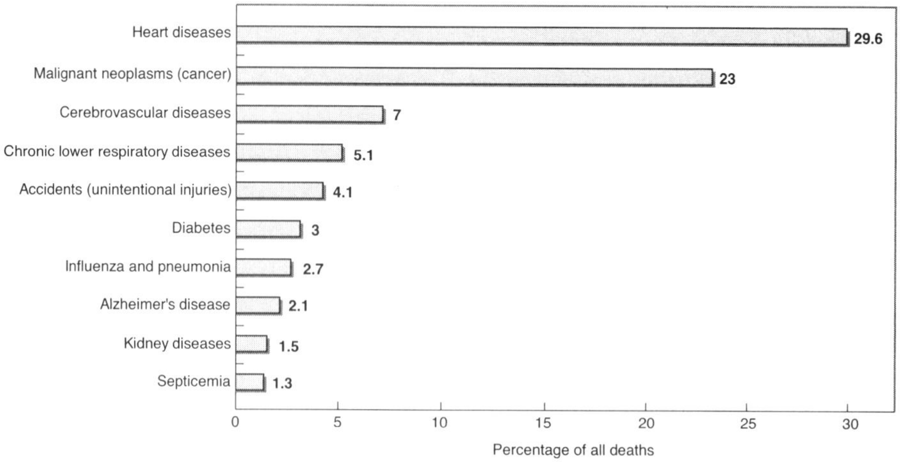

Figure 4-3 Leading Causes of Death in the United States, 2002

Source: National Center for Health Statistics. *Mortality report.* Hyattsville, MD: U.S. Department of Health and Human Services, 2002.

G. *Barriers to eliminating racial disparities in health*
   1. Tuskegee experiment.
   2. Segregation of medical facilities and healthcare providers.
      a. These barriers result in distrust and reluctance to seek care.

H. *Eliminating disparities*
   1. Enforcing Title VI of the Civil Rights Act of 1964, which applies to healthcare providers who receive federal funds or other assistance from the U.S. Department of Health and Human Services (DHHS).
   2. Title VI protects persons of every race (Black, White, Asian), color (skin color regardless of race), and national origin from unlawful discrimination.
   3. *Statement of Title VI*: Recipients of federal financial assistance (hospitals, nursing homes, home health agencies, managed care organizations, health research organizations, physicians, dentists, hospital social workers, as well as other providers who receive federal financial assistance from DHHS) may not on the basis of race, color, or national origin, deny an individ-

ual a service, aid, or other benefit; provide a benefit that is different or provided in a different manner; subject an individual to segregation or separate treatment; restrict an individual in the enjoyment of benefits or privileges; treat an individual differently in determining eligibility; and/or deny a person an opportunity to participate on a planning or advisory board.

4. The DHHS has selected six focus areas in which racial and ethnic minorities experience serious disparities in health access and outcomes: (a) infant mortality, (b) cancer screening and management, (c) cardiovascular disease, (d) diabetes, (e) HIV/AIDS, and (f) immunizations.
5. Ethnic minorities are disproportionately affected by tuberculosis, syphilis, mental illness, and hepatitis. For example, in 2002, 50% of those infected with Hepatitis B were Asian Americans and Pacific Islanders. Black teenagers and young adults become infected with Hepatitis B three to four times more often than those who are White.
6. Designing interventions to address these conditions is imperative for health disparities elimination.

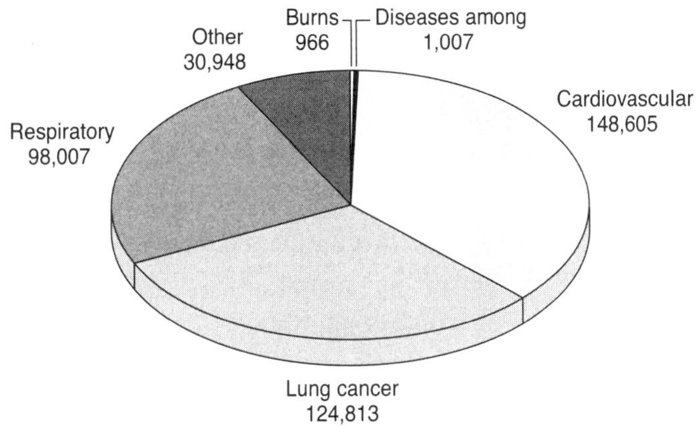

Figure 4-4 Major Diseases Caused by Smoking and Estimated Annual Number of Deaths, 1995–1999

Source: Morbidity and Mortality Weekly Report 51(14): 300–303 (2002).

III. Health Surveys and Behavior Interventions to Promote Health and Prevent Diseases

A. Health surveys serve to gather information on health behaviors, including factors that influence, measure, or are affected by an individual's health.

B. Health surveys are essential for the understanding of how psychological, behavioral, and social factors interact to define health risk behaviors and health.

C. Health surveys serve as important source of information for public health professionals, healthcare policy makers, private healthcare providers, and healthcare consumers concerned with planning, implementing, and evaluating health-related programs and policies.

D. Health surveys may be classified according to: (1) characteristics of environment (political, cultural, social, economic, and physical), (2) population characteristics (demographics, resources, attitudes, knowledge, behavior—acts and reactions), (3) healthcare system characteristics (organizations, programs, insurers, professionals), (4) health status (physical, mental, social), (5) services utilization (type, site, purpose, time interval), (6) expenditures (total, out-of-pocket), and (7) satisfaction status (overall, general, visit-specific).

E. Examples of health surveys that serve as sources of health data include:

1. National Health Interview Survey (NHIS); conducted by the National Center for Health Statistics (NCHS).
    a. The National Health Interview Survey (NHIS) is the leading source of health information on the civilian, noninstitutionalized population in the United States.
    b. NHIS has been conducted annually since 1957 by the National Center for Health Statistics of the Centers for Disease Control and Prevention (CDC).
    c. In-person interviews of the NHIS core questionnaire are used to collect data on demographic, socioeconomic, and healthcare service access characteristics as well as health-related information on everyone in the household.

2. Behavioral Risk Factor Surveillance System (BRFSS); provides state-specific information about issues such as asthma, diabetes, healthcare access, alcohol use, hypertension, obesity, cancer screening, nutrition and physical activity, tobacco use, and more.
   a. The BRFSS is the world's largest, ongoing telephone health survey system, tracking health conditions and risk behaviors in the United States yearly since 1984.
   b. It is conducted by the 50 state health departments as well as those in the District of Columbia, Puerto Rico, Guam, and the U.S. Virgin Islands, with support from the CDC.
3. Health survey: operational steps in design and conduct.
   a. Conceptualization of the topic for survey.
   b. Relating survey design to the objectives of the survey.
   c. Variable ascertainment.
   d. Reflection on the relationship between variables.
   e. Selecting data collection method.
   f. Sampling procedure.
   g. Research question formulation.
   h. Questionnaire formulation.
   i. Survey conduct or performance including monitoring and data safety.
   j. Data cleaning and editing.
   k. Analysis planning and performance (prescreening analysis and hypothesis specific analysis).
   l. Results interpretation.
   m. Report preparation.
4. Behavioral intervention research involves the notion that behavior can be changed.
   a. Interventions to address risky behaviors such as smoking cessation, poor dietary patterns, and physical inactivity have been shown to be efficacious.
   b. These studies have utilized standard methodology that determine efficacy of intervention studies. The translation

of these interventions from efficacy in the trial to effectiveness in the community settings involve the understanding of the following:

1. Which location or agent would work best in the implementation?
2. How many people would choose to use a program that has not been fully evaluated?

5. The basis of behavioral intervention is the consistent indication of behavior change.
   a. Behavioral interventions can successfully teach new behavior:
      1. Behavioral interventions can successfully attenuate risky behaviors.
      2. Maintaining behavior over time, however, is a greater challenge.
      3. Short-term changes in behavior are encouraging, but improved health outcomes will often require prolonged interventions and lengthy follow-up.
      4. Intervention studies are needed to evaluate the efficacy and effectiveness of modifying health risk behaviors.
   b. Intervention studies should span the breadth of all phases of clinical trials, from feasibility studies to randomized double-blinded studies.
   c. Intervention should include all levels of participants, from individual to family, community, and society.
   d. Behavioral and psychosocial interventions should be long term for optimal outcome.
   e. Individual behavior, family interactions, community and workplace relationships and resources, and public policy all contribute to health and influence behavior change.
   f. Interventions at multiple levels (individual, family, community, society) are more likely to sustain behavioral change.

g. Interventions should address psychosocial factors associated with health status, such as access to healthy food and safe places to exercise, as well as individual behavior.
h. Changes are necessary for improvement and maintenance of population health:
    1. Social factors.
    2. Policies.
    3. Norms.

6. *Analysis consideration*:
    a. Research studies, which are based on sample, make inference about the truth in the overall population.
    b. Some of the commonly used designs in studying health-risk behaviors include cross-sectional, or group comparison, longitudinal, and experimental designs.
    c. Essential to longitudinal design is predictive criteria, implying the prediction of changes over time.
    d. *Concerns about longitudinal design*:
        1. Variations in the health indicator may be affected by other external factors in the environment.
        2. Changes in the questions in the successive waves of study could introduce errors in detecting true changes in these indicators over time.
        3. Improvement in diagnostic and treatment modalities or techniques for a selected illness can lead to a higher survival rate, thus a higher prevalence of the disease, over time.
    e. *Multiple regression* procedures may be used when two or more interval-level measures serve as predictors of some normally distributed interval-level dependent variable.
    f. In this model, the regression coefficient for any particular independent or explanatory variable (X_1) represents the change in the response or dependent variable (Y) associated

with a one-unit change in X_1, while controlling for or maintaining other predictors (X_2, X_3, etc.) at constant.

g. *Assumptions*:
   1. The dependent variable should be normally distributed around the prediction line.
   2. All variables are interval, or ratio-scaled.
h. *A two-way analysis of variance*:
   1. An *F*-test statistic can be used to summarize the difference in the variances between the groups on the dependent variable (Y).
   2. The greater the variance between the groups, compared with the variance within the groups, the more likely it is that the differences in X between the groups are statistically significant.
i. *The chi-square statistic* is often used in behavioral data to test for relationships between variables. This procedure is based on the null hypothesis of no association or independence.
   1. Nonparametric procedure involving nominal data.
   2. Examines the difference between the distribution that is observed compared with the distribution that would be expected, assuming the variables are not related.
   3. The less the variance between the observed and expected, the less support there is for the null hypothesis that there is no relationship between the variable in the particular sample.
   4. The purpose of hypothesis testing is to permit generalizations from a sample to the population from which the sample came from (source population). Therefore, hypothesis testing confirms or negates the assertion that the observed findings did not occur by chance alone but rather occurred because of a true or

factual association between the outcome and independent variables.

5. Whether parametric or nonparametric technique of analysis, two types of errors can occur from a study. (1) type I error or alpha error occurs when a significant association is found when indeed there is no association—false positive error, implying the rejection of a TRUE NULL hypothesis, and (2) type II or beta error occurs when one wrongly concludes that there is no significant association, when indeed there is one—false negative, implying the rejection of a TRUE ALTERNATIVE hypothesis.
6. *p* value or alpha level refers to the probability of type I error. Simply, *p* value is a measure of the strength of the evidence provided by the data in favor of the null hypothesis. By convention, the alpha level is set at 0.05 (5% error acceptance). Therefore, if the *p* value is < 0.05 (alpha level), then the evidence against the null hypothesis is strong enough for one to reject it and claim that the observed finding is significant.
7. *p* value limitations: (a) Gives no information about the strength/magnitude of association.
   (b) May be statistically significant but clinically irrelevant or unimportant.
8. 95% Confidence Interval provides information on the magnitude of the association as well as the precision, thus furnishing one with a range of values to interpret the implications of the result.

IV. Health Theories and Health Beliefs

A. *Definitions*

1. *Belief*: Refers to the appraisal of the relationship between some object, action, or idea and some attitude of that

object, action, or idea. Beliefs may develop from direct or indirect experience.

2. *Attitude*: Refers to a relatively stable set of beliefs, feelings, and behavioral tendencies in relation to someone or something.

B. *Health theories and models*: The theories and models used to account for this change include:

1. *Health belief model (HBM)* (developed in 1966 by Rosenstock, a psychologist)
    a. This model maintains that when beliefs affect behavior change, several factors must support a belief before change occurs:
        1. Perceived seriousness of the health problem.
        2. Perceived susceptibility to the health problem.
        3. Cues to action, which implies the influence of direct and indirect cues in making change.
2. *Theory of reasoned action (TRA)*
    a. Proposed by Fishbein (1975) and Ajzen (1981) in an attempt to establish a relationship among beliefs, attitudes, intentions, and behaviors.
    b. TRA is based on two assumptions: (1) humans are rational animals who possess the ability to process and use the information available for them, and (2) humans use the information they process to achieve a reasonable behavioral decision.
    c. According to TRA, the determinant of a person's behavior is his intention to either perform or not to perform the specific behavior.
        1. Due to the difficulties of always determining a person's intention, the theory of reasoned action specified two conceptually independent factors that, interacting together and weighted for the relative importance of each, determine intention (Fishbein & Ajzen, 1975; Ajzen & Madden, 1986).

2. The attitude toward the behavior (A_B) means a personal factor that considers the degree to which a person has positive or negative attitudes about evaluating a specific behavior.

d. Simply, behaviors result from our intention to perform actions.

e. The subjective norm (SN) is a social factor that refers to the apprehended social pressure to either perform or not to perform the behavior in question.

f. Simply, persons are influenced by the approval or disapproval of close friends, loved ones, and social groups.

3. *The theory of planned behavior (TPB)*

a. Adds to the theory of reasoned action the concept of perceived control over the opportunities, resources, and skills necessary to perform a behavior.

b. The concept of perceived behavioral control is similar to the concept of self-efficacy, implying individual's perception of his or her ability to perform the behavior.

c. Perceived behavioral control over opportunities, resources, and skills necessary to perform a behavior is believed to be a critical aspect of behavior change processes.

4. *Transtheoretical model (TTM) of health behavior change*

a. Serves as the basis for developing effective interventions to promote health behavior change.

b. Proposed by Prochaska and DiClemente (1983); Prochaska, DiClemente, and Norcross, (1992); and Prochaska and Velicer (1997).

c. TTM is an integrative model of behavior change that describes how people modify a problem behavior or acquire a positive behavior.

d. The central organizing construct of the model is *the stages of change* and includes a series of independent variables:

the *processes of change* and a series of outcome measures, including the *decisional balance* and the *temptation scales.*

e. Interventions based on the TTM potentially have both a high efficacy and a high recruitment rate, thus dramatically increasing the potential impact on entire populations of individuals with behavioral health risks.

f. The stages of change as proposed in the model are as follows:

   1. *Pre-contemplation* is the stage in which people are not intending to take action in the foreseeable future, usually measured as the next six months.
   2. *Contemplation* is the stage in which people are intending to change in the next six months.
   3. *Preparation* is the stage in which people are intending to take action in the immediate future, usually measured as the next month.
   4. *Action* is the stage in which people have made specific overt modifications in their lifestyles within the past six months.
   5. *Maintenance* is the stage in which people are working to prevent relapse but do not apply change processes as frequently as do people in action.

5. *Social learning theory (social cognitive theory)*

   a. Proposes that behavior change is affected by environmental influences, personal factors, and attributes of the behavior itself.
   b. Each may affect or be affected by either of the other two, with the central tenet of social cognitive theory being the concept of self-efficacy.
   c. A person must believe in his or her capability to perform the behavior (i.e., the person must possess self-efficacy) and must perceive an incentive to do so (i.e., the person's positive expectations from performing the behavior must outweigh the negative expectations).

d. A person must value the outcomes or consequences that he or she believes will occur as a result of performing a specific behavior or action.
e. Outcomes may be classified as having immediate benefits (e.g., feeling energized following physical activity) or long-term benefits (e.g., experiencing improvements in cardiovascular health as a result of physical activity).
    1. Because these expected outcomes are filtered through a person's expectations or perceptions of being able to perform the behavior in the first place, self-efficacy is believed to be the single most important characteristic that determines a person's behavior change.
    2. Self-efficacy can be increased in several ways, among them are providing clear instructions, providing the opportunity for skill development or training, and modeling the desired behavior.

6. *Ecological theory of behavior change*
    a. Most theories and models of behavior change tend to emphasize individual behavior change process and pay little attention to sociocultural and physical environmental influences on behavior.
    b. Ecological approaches to increasing participation in an intervention focuses on sociocultural and environmental influences on behavior.
    c. These approaches emphasize the creation of supportive environments as well as the development of personal skills and the reorientation of health services.
    d. An underlying theme of ecological perspectives is that the most effective interventions occur on multiple levels.
    e. A model has been proposed that encompasses several levels of influences on health behaviors: intrapersonal factors, interpersonal and group factors, institutional factors, community factors, and public policy.

f. Similarly, another model has three levels (individual, organizational, and governmental) in four settings (schools, worksites, healthcare institutions, and communities).
g. Interventions that simultaneously influence these multiple levels and multiple settings may be expected to lead to greater and longer-lasting changes and maintenance of existing health-promoting habits.
h. This is a promising area for the design of future intervention research to promote physical activity.

7. *Relapse prevention model*
   a. Focuses on factors that contribute to relapse, including negative emotional or physiologic states, limited coping skills, social pressure, interpersonal conflict, limited social support, low motivation, high-risk situations, and stress.
   b. Principles include identifying high-risk situations for relapse (e.g., change in season) and developing appropriate solutions (e.g., finding a place to walk inside during the winter).

Table 4-2 Similarities and Differences of the Behavior Change Theories and Models

Theory/Model	Description
Health belief	Highlights the role of the perceived outcomes of behavior, although different terms are used for this construct, including perceived benefits and barriers
Social cognitive/ planned behavior	Highlights the role of the perceived outcomes of behavior, although different terms are used for this construct, including perceived benefits and barriers and outcome expectations

Table 4-2 Similarities and Differences of the Behavior Change Theories and Models *(continued)*

Theory/Model	Description
Reasoned action and planned behavior	Emphasizes the influence of perceptions of control over behavior; this influence is given labels such as self-efficacy (health belief model, social cognitive theory) and perceived behavioral control
Ecologic model	Emphasizes social support, interpersonal and environmental influences

C. Some similarities can be noted among the behavioral and social science theories and models used to understand and enhance health behaviors such as physical activity.

D. Most of the theories and models, however, do not address the influence of the environment on health behavior.

V. Behavioral Risk Factors in Major Diseases [Chronic Diseases, Cancer, Maternal and Child Health, Infant Mortality, Infectious Diseases Including Sexually Transmitted Infections (STIs) and HIV, and Conditions (Obesity, Pregnancy)]

A. *Predisposing, enabling, and reinforcing factors*

1. Predisposing factors in disease, disability, and injury include: (a) knowledge, (b) beliefs, (c) values, (d) attitudes, (e) culture, (f) socio-demographics (gender, age, income, education, marital status), and (g) access and utilization of the healthcare system.
2. Enabling factors in health include: (a) skills and capabilities; (b) adequate support and resources; (c) health resources availability; (d) community and governmental support, prioritization, and commitment to health; (e) health-related skills; (f) physical, mental, and emotional capabilities; (g) time and financial resources; and (h) safe areas (environment).
3. Reinforcing factors in health include: (a) family support system; (b) social support network; (c) peer support; (d) employer actions

and policies; (e) health provider cost and access, as well as low cost and utilization of quality health care; (f) access to public health and patient education; and (g) community resources.

4. Outcomes of interaction between predisposing, enabling, and reinforcing factors result in (a) regular health assessment; (b) weight management; (c) improved relationship (inter- and intrapersonal); (d) safer sexual behaviors; (e) safer drug use; (f) improved dietary patterns; (g) stress management and control; (h) improved consumer decisions; and (i) increased physical activities.
5. The outcome of the behavior change given a healthy interaction between predisposing, enabling, and reinforcing factors are reductions in (a) chronic disabilities, (b) STIs, (c) heart diseases, (d) cancer, (e) mortality due to auto accidents, and (f) infant and maternal mortality.

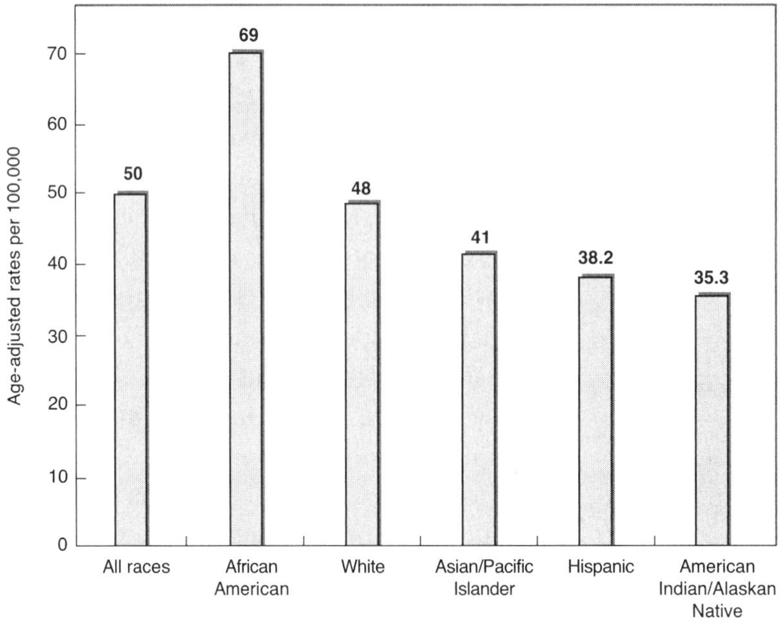

Figure 4-5 Age-Adjusted Mortality Rates per 100,000 Persons by Race/Ethnicity for Cerebrovascular Disease: United States, 2004

Source: Health US, 2006, www.cdc.gov/nchs/data/huso6.pdf#summary, Table 29.

B. *Behavioral risk factors in major diseases and health indicators*
1. Heart disease, malignant neoplasm, and stroke, which are chronic diseases, are the three leading causes of morbidity and mortality in the United States.
2. These conditions are linked with a limited number of health risk behaviors, such as cigarette smoking, poor nutrition, physical inactivity, and underuse of prevention practices.
3. Preventing and reducing the prevalence of health risk behaviors and subsequent morbidity and mortality attributed to chronic diseases remains a major goal of public health.
4. The Healthy People 2010 (HP 2010) objectives aim to reduce the impact of high-risk behaviors and increase use of preventive services.

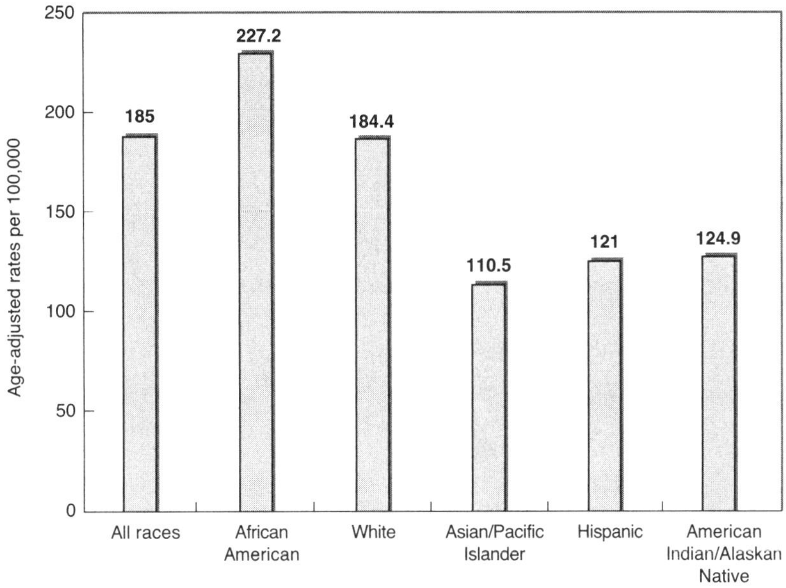

Figure 4-6 Age-Adjusted Mortality Rates per 100,000 Persons by Race/Ethnicity for Malignant Neoplasm: United States, 2004

Source: Health US, 2006, www.cdc.gov/nchs/data/huso6.pdf#summary, Table 29.

C. *Basic notions in health risk behaviors*
   1. *Risk or predisposing* factors to disease and disabilities are both modifiable and nonmodifiable.
   2. *Modifiable risk factors* are those that are controllable or treatable such as lifestyle and the lowering of serum cholesterol or glucose level by treatment compliance.
   3. *Nonmodifiable risk factors* are factors predisposing to disease that are uncontrollable such as age, gender, and race/ethnicity.
   4. Modifiable risk factors present a great potential for the control, reduction, and elimination of diseases.
   5. Behavior changes that affect lifestyle remain the hallmark of diseases that are associated with modifiable risks such as chronic diseases, chronic disabilities, and infectious diseases.

D. *Health risk behaviors (risk factors) associated with heart disease* (first leading cause of mortality in the United States, representing 29.5% of the total causes of death in 2002); modifiable risk factors are (health risk behaviors):
   1. High blood cholesterol, mainly disproportional balance between HDL and LDL, resulting in higher ratio of LDL to HDL.
   2. High blood pressure.
   3. Smoking—accounts for nearly 30% of all deaths due to heart disease, as well as the leading predisposing factor to death in the United States (18.1%).
   4. Physical inactivity.
   5. Overweight and obesity.
   6. Diabetes.

E. *Health risk behaviors (risk factors) associated with stroke* (third leading cause of death in the United States, representing 6.9% of the total cause of death in 2002); modifiable risk factors are (health risk behaviors):
   1. Smoking—active and passive.
   2. Alcohol use.

3. Obesity.
4. Uncontrolled high blood pressure.
5. Physical inactivity.

F. *Health risk behaviors (behavioral risk factors) associated with major malignant neoplasm* (second leading cause of death in the United States, accounting for 22.9% of all deaths in 2002); modifiable risk factors (health risk behaviors):
1. Obesity and overweight (colon, endometrial, breast cancers).
2. Smoking—active and passive (renal, lung, oral cavity neoplasm).
3. Physical inactivity.
4. High-fat diet.
5. Alcohol consumption (oral cavity neoplasm).
6. Excessive exposure to ultraviolet radiation (sunlight).

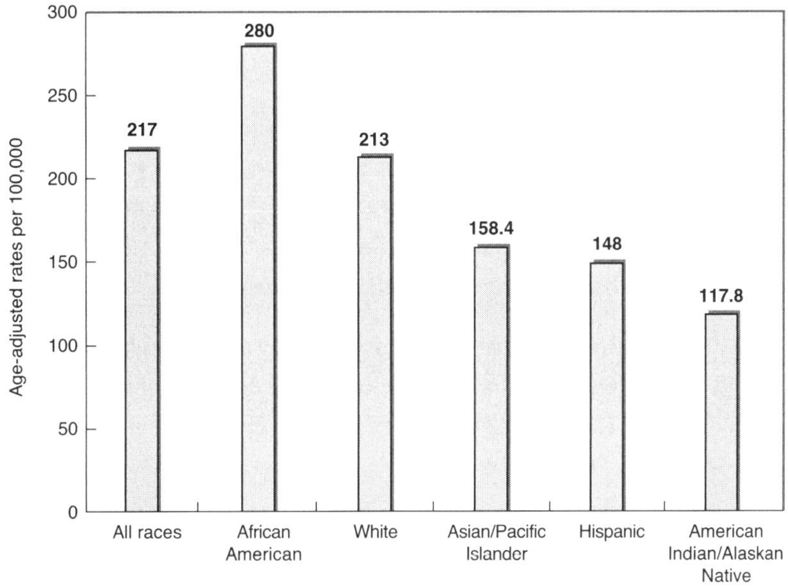

Figure 4-7 Age-Adjusted Mortality Rates per 100,000 Persons by Race/Ethnicity for Heart Disease: United States, 2004

Source: Health US, 2006, www.cdc.gov/nchs/data/huso6.pdf#summary, Table 29.

G. *Diabetes mellitus*: Health risk behaviors include:
   1. Physical inactivity leading to obesity.
   2. Poor dietary habits.
   3. Alcohol.
   4. Smoking.
   5. Obesity.

H. *Hypertension*: Health risk behaviors include:
   1. Physical inactivity.
   2. High sodium intake.
   3. Impaired coping skills—stress management.
   4. High-fat/lipid diet.
   5. Lack of rest (inadequate sleep).
   6. Excessive alcohol consumption.
   7. Smoking.

I. *HIV/AIDS*: Health risk behaviors include:
   1. Drug and alcohol use.
   2. Unprotected sex.
   3. Multiple sexual partners.
   4. Lack of risk perception and self-efficacy.
   5. Exchange of sex for drugs or money.

J. Inadequate health monitoring/screening and lack health education are health risk behaviors that are associated with the preceding illustrative health conditions.

VI. Health Promotion Components and Levels of Disease Prevention

A. *Health promotion* involves the following components:
   1. *Educational*: provision of information about risk behaviors and their consequences.
   2. *Organizational*: provision of programs and services that encourage participation and establish social support system.
   3. *Environmental*: provision of regulatory mechanisms to govern behavior and support behavior change or modification.

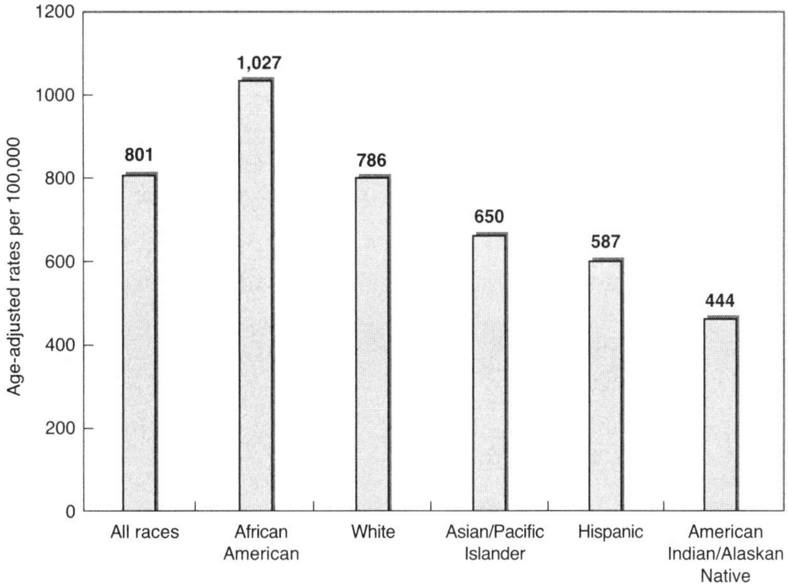

Figure 4-8 Age-Adjusted Mortality Rates per 100,000 Persons by Race/Ethnicity for All Causes of Death: United States, 2004

Source: Health US, 2006, www.cdc.gov/nchs/data/huso6.pdf#summary, Table 29.

4. *Financial*: provision of incentive such as monetary to maintain healthful behaviors.

B. *Disease prevention* involves three basic levels:
1. *Primary prevention* refers to risk reduction and health problems avoidance in the first place.
2. *Secondary prevention* refers to the provision of intervention to reduce or eliminate risk or predisposing behaviors before the progression to clinical or overt disease state.
3. *Tertiary prevention* refers to the provision of treatment or rehabilitation after the event has already occurred in order to reduce its complications (e.g., stroke rehabilitation).

REVIEW QUESTIONS (MULTIPLE CHOICE)

Directions: Each question below contains multiple suggested responses. Select the *one best* response to each question.

1. The bio-psychosocial model of health, which focuses on the multifactorial causes of disease, could be applied to which of the following conditions as an attempt to understand their ethio-pathogenesis?

- **a.** Cardiovascular disorders
- **b.** Cancer
- **c.** Diabetes
- **d.** a and c only
- **e.** All of the above

2. An investigator is interested in a behavioral intervention that will increase self-efficacy in the participants. Under which of the following conditions will self-efficacy be an effective intervention model in reducing the behavioral risk and maintain healthful behaviors?

- **a.** Smoking
- **b.** Sexual behavior
- **c.** Drug abuse
- **d.** b and c only
- **e.** All of the above

3. The potential for biological, chemical, and nuclear agents to be used in a terrorist attack has received wide publicity in the United States since the attacks on September 11, 2001. However, the role of public health, through behavioral sciences, in attempting to understand the present terrorists threats and concerns with the immediate and long-term behavioral consequences of terrorism remain unclear. As a public health professional, what will you consider to be the *main* purpose(s) of terrorism?

- **a.** Instill fear in the population
- **b.** Change the behavior of governments
- **c.** Compress mortality
- **d.** a and b only
- **e.** All of the above

4. A survey study conducted to examine the emerging risk factors in diabetes mellitus in New-town, No-State, revealed excessive inactivity as one of the exposure (independent/predictor) variables. As a public health professional, you are expected to implement an intervention to increase physical activities in this population. The strategies for this behavior change will include:

- **a.** Individual
- **b.** Group
- **c.** Community
- **d.** Technology-based
- **e.** All of the above

5. Social and economic factors are major determinants of health. Which of the following statement(s) is (are) *correct* regarding the observed role of this factor in disease progression and prognosis?

- **a.** The quality of the social environment is worse where financial deprivation is greatest, such as the inner cities
- **b.** The ill effects due to absolute poverty—meaning societies in which there is a wide gap between the rich and the poor—suffer additional social problems, for instance, through high rates of violence, crime, and truancy
- **c.** People with good social networks live longer, are at reduced risk of coronary heart disease, are less likely to report being depressed, are

less likely to suffer a recurrence of cancer, and are less susceptible to infectious illness than those with poor networks

d. a and b only
e. All of the above

6. The life expectancy gained in the U.S. population has been attributed to behavior changes at the population level toward tobacco cessation practices. This resulted in a dramatic decrease in heart diseases and stroke. Tobacco remains the leading predisposing factor to death in the United States, accounting for 18.1% of the total predisposing factors and conditions associated with death. Which of the following health condition(s) is (are) associated with smoking?

a. Lung, mouth, and throat cancers
b. Chronic obstructive pulmonary disease
c. Renal cancer
d. a and c only
e. All of the above

7. The ecologic model of health behavior proposes the role of social environment in the implementation of an effective health promotion and disease prevention program. As a public health professional, the City Health Department wishes to reduce the obesity epidemic among inner-city Hispanic males by using the ecologic model. Which of the following stages will be *essential* in your implementation?

a. Intrapersonal factors
b. Interpersonal factors
c. Institutional factors
d. Community factors
e. Public policy
f. a, c, and e only
g. All of the above

8. During the past three decades, a great deal of research has been focused on how to increase people's self-efficacy, thereby helping to motivate them to practice healthy behaviors. As a proponent of this model of behavior change, which of the following examples would you consider *adequate* in increasing self-efficacy?

- **a.** Previous successful performance
- **b.** Role-modeling
- **c.** Small-group exercise
- **d.** Skills practice
- **e.** All of the above
- **f.** None of the above

9. Studies on psychological and social factors that influence health have consistently implicated stress and social support in the outcome of disease and mortality. Which of the following statements support the role played by stress in disease prognosis and mortality?

- **a.** Widows and widowers tend to have an unusually high risk of dying soon after the death of their spouse
- **b.** Mortality rates of survivors are 40% to 50% higher during the six months after the death of a spouse relative to the mortality of married people of the same age
- **c.** People who lose their jobs are 50% to 70% more likely to present with angina symptoms, compared to their employed counterparts of the same age and similar socio-demographics
- **d.** a and c only
- **e.** All of the above

10. Race and ethnicity are consistently shown to influence disease prevalence and mortality in the United States, and ethnic minorities, particularly Blacks, tend to be disproportionately affected and bear the burden of most diseases in the nation. Because race/ethnicity is a complex phenomenon, which of the following demographic variations may explain the observed burden of morbidity and mortality of the Blacks relative to Whites?

- **a.** Income
- **b.** Education
- **c.** Occupation
- **d.** a and c only
- **e.** All of the above

11. Social support network has been found to be strongly associated with an individual's health status and risk of dying. This association is observed to be true for both genders regardless of socioeconomic status. Because the absence of social support or contact has been associated with increase in coronary heart disease, pregnancy complications, and prematurity and infant mortality, which of the following statements provide a possible explanation to the observed associations?

- **a.** Social contact is effective in stress buffering
- **b.** Relaxation may be achieved through social contacts and social support networks
- **c.** Social contact increases adrenal gland secretion, releasing excessive dopamine and norepinephrine, thus reducing stress
- **d.** Social contact may potentiate the immune responsiveness, thus serving as a protective mechanism for tissue inflammation and repair
- **e.** a, b, and d only

12. The health belief model of behavior change assumes that humans act in rational ways and are more likely to change behavior when confronted with a threat. If you are assigned to a breast cancer prevention program (BCPP) and wish to use this model in promoting breast self-examination among Asian-American women, which of the following factors will you consider in your implementation of this model?

- **a.** The extent to which Asian-American women feel vulnerable to breast cancer
- **b.** The perceived severity of breast cancer
- **c.** The perceived effectiveness of taking action to prevent or minimize breast cancer as compared to barriers to and costs of taking such an action
- **d.** All of the above
- **e.** None of the above

13. Interventions to address risky behaviors such as smoking cessation, poor dietary patterns, and physical inactivity have been shown to be efficacious. These studies have utilized standard methodology that determine efficacy of intervention studies. As a public health professional, if you wish to replicate or translate these proven interventions to your community in determining their effectiveness, which of the following aspects of community-based intervention will you consider?

- **a.** Population that might benefit most from the intervention
- **b.** Which location or agent would work best in the implementation
- **c.** How many people would choose to use a program that has not been fully evaluated
- **d.** All of the above
- **e.** None of the above

14. The basis of behavioral intervention is the consistent indication of behavior change. Which of the following statements is *inaccurate* concerning behavior change?

- **a.** Behavioral interventions can successfully teach new behavior
- **b.** Behavioral interventions are solely designed to potentiate risky behaviors
- **c.** Behavioral interventions can successfully attenuate risky behaviors
- **d.** Maintaining behavior over time, however, is a greater challenge
- **e.** Short-term changes in behavior are encouraging, but improved health outcomes will often require prolonged interventions and lengthy follow-up

15. Research efforts to elucidate the mechanisms by which social and psychological factors influence health are essential to health promotions and disease prevention. Which of the following is *correct* regarding behavioral intervention?

- **a.** Intervention studies are needed to evaluate the efficacy and effectiveness of modifying health risk behaviors
- **b.** Intervention studies should span the breadth of all phases of clinical trials, from feasibility studies to randomized double-blinded studies
- **c.** Intervention should include all levels of participants, from individual to family, community, and society
- **d.** All of the above
- **e.** None of the above

16. All of the following are correct concerning intervention strategy *except*:

- **a.** Concurrent intervention at multiple levels should not be encouraged as this will not lead to the promotion of healthy behaviors
- **b.** Behavioral and psychosocial interventions should be long term for optimal outcome

c. Individual behavior, family interactions, community and workplace relationships, resources, and public policy all contribute to health and influence behavior change
d. Interventions at multiple levels (individual, family, community, society) are more likely to sustain behavioral change
e. Interventions should address psychosocial factors associated with health status, such as access to healthy food and safe places to exercise, as well as individual behavior

17. Changing unhealthy behavior is not simply a matter of "willpower." Individual behavior has biological underpinnings and consequences and is influenced by the social and psychological contexts in which it occurs. Which of the following changes are *necessary* for improvement and maintenance of population health?

a. Social factors
b. Policies
c. Norms
d. All of the above
e. a and c only

18. Obesity is next to tobacco in terms of population's burden of disease. This condition is dramatically increasing and has become epidemic in the United States. All of the following health risk behaviors or conditions are linked to this epidemic, *except*:

a. Excessive caloric intake
b. Inadequate physical activity
c. Diabetes
d. Birth defects
e. Osteoporosis

19. Interventions at individual and group levels have been conducted to reduce HIV risk behaviors among the most vulnerable populations at highest risk in the United States. In spite of these interventions, African-American women remain the fastest growing segment of incident AIDS cases. Obviously, new research studies are needed to provide intervention at individual, family, community, and society levels. As an HIV/AIDS interventionist, which of the following factors will you consider as HIV/AIDS-related behavior to incorporate into your model in reducing HIV risky behaviors?

a. Knowledge
b. Subjective norms
c. Perceived risk
d. Self-efficacy
e. All of the above

20. Smoking behavior tends to follow some socio-demographic patterns. Which of the following findings or statements support such observed patterns?

a. The prevalence of smoking among blue-collar workers is higher compared with white-collar workers
b. Compared with Whites or Blacks, American Indians and Alaskan Natives smoke at much higher rates
c. The prevalence rate of smoking is higher among men with less than high school education compared with male and female college students of the same age
d. All of the above
e. None of the above

21. The Behavioral Risk Factor Surveillance System (BRFSS) is a source of data for health risk behaviors in chronic and infectious diseases. The Youth Risk Behavior Survey is another source of data for health risk factors. This dataset characterizes the prevalence of selected health risk behaviors among adolescents aged 12 to 19 years who do and do not attend school. Which of the following findings serve to support the role of education in health risk behaviors?

a. In-school adolescents are significantly more likely to have reported "always" using safety belts while riding in a car or truck, relative to out-of-school adolescents
b. In-school adolescents are less likely to report driving under the influence of alcohol
c. Out-of-school adolescents are significantly less likely to use marijuana or cocaine
d. All of the above
e. None of the above

22. Public health researchers should consider the particular study design being used in their survey and the type of research questions that can be addressed with the design. Some of the commonly used study designs in studying health risk behaviors include cross-sectional (or group comparison), longitudinal, and experimental designs. Essential to longitudinal design is predictive criteria, implying the prediction of changes over time. Which of the following statements is (are) *true* regarding this design (longitudinal)?

a. Variations in the health indicator may be affected by other external factors in the environment
b. Changes in the questions in the successive waves of the study could introduce errors in detecting true changes in these indicators over time
c. Improvement in diagnostic and treatment modalities or techniques for a selected illness can lead to a higher survival, thus a higher prevalence of the disease over time
d. a and b only
e. All of the above

23. Multiple regression procedures may be used when two or more interval-level measures serve as predictors of some normally distributed interval-level dependent variable. In this model, the regression coefficient for any particular independent or explanatory variable (X_1) represents the change in the response or dependent variable (Y) associated with a one-unit change in X_1, while controlling for or maintaining other predictors (X_2, X_3, etc.) at constant. If required to use this predictive model in the analysis of study data, which of the following assumptions are *necessary* for a valid result?

a. The dependent variable should be normally distributed around the prediction line
b. All variables are interval- or ratio-scaled
c. Both of the above
d. None of the above

24. A study was conducted to examine the differences in average cholesterol level of Black and Asian children (X_1), while controlling for poverty status (X_2). If the analytic method used here is the two-way analysis of variance, which of the following statements is (are) *correct* regarding this technique?

a. An *F*-test statistic can be used to summarize the difference in the variances between and within Black and Asian children on the dependent variable (Y)
b. The greater the variance between Black and Asian children, compared with the variance within Black children and the variance within Asian children, the more likely it is that the differences in cholesterol level between Black and Asian children are statistically significant
c. Both of the above
d. None of the above

25. The chi-square statistic is often used in behavioral data to test for relationships between variables. This procedure is based on the null hypothesis of no association or independence. Which of the following statements is (are) *correct* regarding this analytic technique?

a. It is a nonparametric procedure involving nominal data
b. It examines the difference between the distribution that is observed and the distribution that would be expected, assuming the variables are not related
c. The less the variance between the observed and expected, the less support there is for the null hypothesis that there is no relationship between the variable in the particular sample
d. a and c only
e. All of the above

26. Obesity intervention often utilized community trials to increase physical activity. These trials are usually part of a "healthy heart" program and incorporate social and environmental measures, including public service announcements about physical activity and total well-being. This approach in terms of health behavior model is *best* described as the:

a. Transtheoretical model
b. Health belief model
c. Social support model
d. Ecologic model
e. Information, motivation and skill building model

27. Recent investigations regarding the overall health of the U.S. population indicated improvement over the past few decades. However, health disparities among racial and ethnic minorities have persisted. Which of the following statements support these findings?

a. Life expectancy in 2001 was 77.7 for Whites and 72.2 for Blacks
b. African-American women in 2006 represent an estimated 70% of total incident AIDS cases among women
c. Infant mortality rate for Blacks in 2001 was 2.3 times higher than that of Whites
d. All of the above
e. None of the above

28. Effective behavior intervention transcends the individual and involves family, groups, and public policy. Which of the following illustrates the influence of policy in behavior change?

- **a.** Raising tobacco taxes
- **b.** A company's reduction of the price of cigarettes
- **c.** Restrictions on advertising and promotion
- **d.** a and c only
- **e.** None of the above

29. Infant mortality has declined in the United States over the past decade due to improved socioeconomic status, housing, nutrition, immunization, clean water and pasteurized milk, antibiotics, and improved prenatal and delivery care. The specific causes differ by race, with the leading cause of infant mortality for Whites being congenital anomalies and for Blacks, prematurity and low birth weight. Which of the following factors may help explain the variation in the race-specific etiology of infant mortality?

- **a.** Lower socioeconomic status of African Americans
- **b.** Out-of-wedlock birth of African Americans
- **c.** Young maternal age and low maternal education of African Americans
- **d.** Maternal alcohol consumption of White Americans
- **e.** All of the above

30. One of the conditions for the efficacy of a behavioral intervention is the duration of intervention and the immunization of loss to follow-up or retention. Which of these intervention models of behavior change explicitly claims a high degree of retention of subjects?

- **a.** Health belief
- **b.** Information motivation and skill building
- **c.** Transtheoretical
- **d.** Theory of reasoned action
- **e.** Social cognitive

ANNOTATED ANSWERS

1. The correct answer is **E** (bio-psychosocial aspect of health and illness).

2. The correct answer is **E** (intervention model and risk reduction).

3. The correct answer is **D** (behavioral and psychosocial aspect of terrorism).

4. The correct answer is **E** (behavioral and social factors in health).

5. The correct answer is **E** (socio-economic and social class determinant of health).

6. The correct answer is **E** (smoking as a modifiable risk factor in disease causation and mortality).

7. The correct answer is **G** (ecologic model of health behavior).

8. The correct answer is **E** (psychosocial model of behavior).

9. The correct answer is **E** (influence of stress and social support on health behavior).

10. The correct answer is **E** (racial disparities in health).

11. The correct answer is **E** (social support system and health outcomes).

12. The correct answer is **D** (health belief model of behavior change).

13. The correct answer is **D** (research translation—efficacy to effectiveness).

14. The correct answer is **B** (behavioral interventions).

15. The correct answer is **D** (behavioral interventions).

16. The correct answer is **A** (behavioral intervention strategies).

17. The correct answer is **D** (population health determinants).

18. The correct answer is **E** (obesity epidemic and health consequences).

19. The correct answer is **E** (disease-specific intervention).

20. The correct answer is **D** (socio-demographic influence on smoking).

21. The correct answer is **D** (influence of education on youth health risk behavior).

22. The correct answer is **E** (health survey study—longitudinal design).

23. The correct answer is **C** (multiple regression analysis).

24. The correct answer is **C** (analysis of variance—ANOVA).

25. The correct answer is **E** (nonparametric analysis).

26. The correct answer is **D** (health behavior models).

27. The correct answer is **D** (health disparities).

28. The correct answer is **D** (government role/policy in health promotion).

29. The correct answer is **E** (racial variation in cause-specific infant mortality).

30. The correct answer is **C** (behavior change model).

Chapter 5

Environmental Sciences in Public Health

Larry Holmes, Jr., and Jennifer Thompson

OVERVIEW

Public health originated from the initiative or effort to provide clean drinking water and avoid contaminated food. The *environmental* aspect of public health focused on these two aspects by controlling water and food safety, thus preventing diarrheal illnesses and mortality across human populations. With the modern environment, public health initiatives in this direction underwent a dramatic transition. Growing industries and the use of coal and fossil fuel resulted in increased levels of carbon dioxide emissions, increased global warming, and the contributions of environmental air pollutants and their interactions with O_2 at lower atmospheric levels, thus resulting in higher ozone levels. In addition, the growth in industries and manufacturing has generated millions of tons of toxic heavy metals (manganese, nickel, chromium, cadmium), some of which are carcinogenic to humans, thus increasing human risk of cancer. Solid-waste generation and impaired disposal processes have increased during the past three decades as well as exposure to ionizing radiation. The health effects of these environmental air, water, and soil pollutants contribute to the deteriorating health of the human population. The current role of the environmental sciences is to identify the environmental or toxic substances through risk assessment (and risk characterization), continue to evaluate the safety level of exposure of these substances, encourage the development of health policies to minimize their risk, and develop interventions to prevent exposure to these pollutants (air, water, heavy metals, biologic, solid hazardous wastes, ionizing radiation). Environmental health is challenged with the explosive human population, given the degradation of water sources and increasing food scarcity as a result of deforestation and poor agricultural productivity. Thus, generating enough food to sustain the expanding human population remains the challenge of environmental public health in the nearest future.

This chapter reviews the basic principles in risk assessment, environmental toxins as toxic substances, and the impacts of those substances on human health or the health effects on the biologic system.

I. **Environmental Sciences and Public Health**

A. Historically, the role of environmental sciences in public health had been reducing and eliminating the incidence and prevalence of diseases caused and spread by contaminated water and food.

B. Besides contaminated food and water, air contamination, radiation, pesticides, noise, motor vehicles, exposure to several occupational chemicals, and global warming present health hazards, and are significant threats of the modern environment.

C. Toxic pollutants [synthetic chemical waste, combustion products (air pollutants), chemical additives in food] act at the cellular level to initiate often irreversible changes that can induce cellular damage and abnormal cellular proliferation.

D. Further examples are exposure to X-rays, organic chemicals, and heavy metals (such as mercury, manganese, chromium, cadmium), which can damage the cell or lead to neoplastic outcomes via uncontrolled cellular proliferation.

E. The interaction of toxic substances in the environment may lead to:

1. Mutation (point mutation, chromosomal aberrations, and change in chromosome numbers).
2. Birth defects (phocomelia, fetal alcohol syndrome).
3. Neoplastic disorders (cancers of various sites).
4. Chronic disease (cardiovascular disease, hypertension, stroke, asthma, COPD).

F. *Environmental sciences as an applied core discipline of public health* presently deals with the identification of toxic pollutants or substances, their mechanisms of disease causation, and application of this knowledge and environmental policies to prevent and control environmental diseases, disabilities, injuries, and health-related events.

G. *Environmental health* deals with the burden of disease attributable to environmental factors.
   1. Cause-and-effect relationships between water, air pollution, and human health have been well established.
   2. Health consequences of other environmental factors and exposures, such as those resulting from climate change and chemicals in the environment, are a result of complex interactions between the environment and humans that are far less understood.
   3. For some chemicals, such as endocrine-disrupting substances, the effects on humans are particularly difficult to unravel, but the impacts on wildlife have been substantial, with implications for human health.
   4. Other chemicals in the environment, the disposal of wastes, and noise continue to generate concerns about their health effects on humans.

H. Vulnerability and exposure, however, vary markedly between different groups and areas, with children and the elderly being particularly at risk.

I. Diseases associated with environmental factors have been well documented. Examples are allergies and asthma; neurotoxic effects of environmental contaminants; environmental factors influencing the onset of puberty; food and fertility; and cancer, heart disease, and obesity associated with risks correlated to environment, diet, and genetic factors.
   1. Outdoor air pollution plays a role in the causation and aggravation of asthma and allergic responses, which are increasingly prevalent diseases, especially in children.

2. Much of the outdoor air penetrates indoors, and as people breathe both, an integrated approach to both outdoor and indoor air pollution is necessary.
3. Transport continues to be a significant contributor to health effects from accidents, air pollution, and noise.

Table 5-1 Types of Mutations

Mutation	Description
Point mutation	Involves a change at the molecular level within a gene Results from deletion or substitution of a base pair—impaired protein formation Most common type of mutation
Chromosomal aberration	Gross structural changes in the chromosome Caused by loss or addition of sizable pieces of a chromosome or reversing of chromosome part May result in lethal mutation
Change in chromosome number	Caused by nondisjunction or paired homologous chromosomes during meiosis

Table 5-2 Teratogens and Their Effects

Teratogens	Teratogenic Effect
Microbes	
Toxoplasmosis	Central nervous system (CNS) abnormalities
Syphilis and herpes simplex type 2	Mental retardation, microcephaly, kidney and liver disorders, brain abnormalities
German measles	Congenital heart defect, deafness and hearing impairment, cataracts
Ionizing radiation	
X-rays	CNS disorders, microcephaly, visual disorders, and mental retardation

Table 5-2 Teratogens and Their Effects *(continued)*

Teratogens	Teratogenic Effect
Drugs and chemicals	
Thalidomide	Phocomelia, or seal-limb, in which a hand or foot is attached directly to the torso without an arm or foot
Dioxin	Structural abnormalities and miscarriage
Dilantin	Heart malformations, cleft palate, mental retardation, microcephaly
Tobacco	Low birth weight, miscarriage, stillbirth
Valporic acid	Spina bifida
Tegison	Cardiovascular abnormalities, ear deformation, hydrocephaly, microcephaly
Accutane	Cardiovascular abnormalities, ear deformation, hydrocephaly, microcephaly
Anesthesia	Miscarriages and structural abnormalities
DES*	Vagina cancer in girls and genital abnormalities in boys
Methyl mercury	Mental retardation, neuro-developmental disorders

*DES = Diethylbesterol

II. Health Hazards and Risk Assessment

A. *Risk* refers to undesirable consequence of a particular activity in relation to the likelihood that it may occur.

B. *Risk assessment* is an estimate of the likelihood of adverse effects that may result from exposure to certain health hazards (e.g., toxic substances in the environment).

C. *Risk management* decisions follow the identification and quantification of risk, which is determined by risk assessments.

D. During the regulatory process, *risk managers* may request that additional risk assessments be conducted to justify the risk management decisions.

E. Risk assessments may be conducted for individual chemicals or for complex mixtures of chemicals. In cases of complex mixtures, such as hazardous waste sites, the process of risk assessment itself becomes quite complex.

F. Basic notions of risk assessment

1. *Hazard* refers to the capability of a substance to cause an adverse effect.
2. *Risk* refers to the probability that the hazard will occur under specific exposure conditions.
3. *Risk assessment* refers to the process by which hazards, exposure, and risk are determined.
4. *Risk management* refers to the process of weighing policy alternatives and selecting the most appropriate regulatory action based on the results of risk assessment and social, economic, and political concerns.
    a. A risk is the chance that an adverse event will happen, multiplied by the extent of the effect.
    b. *Mathematically*, Risk (R) = $F \times E$, where F = frequency of the exposure and E = effect of exposure.
    c. Therefore, risk quantifies the product of the frequency and effect of an exposure (toxic substance).

Table 5-3 Steps in Risk Assessment Process

Step	Process	Description
I	Hazard identification	The health conditions associated with or caused by the pollutants
II	Exposure assessment	The amount of pollutant inhaled or ingested during a specific time period The number exposed
III	Dose-response assessment	The health conditions/problems at different exposure levels/doses
IV	Risk characterization	The extra risk (excess) of the health problems in the exposed population

G. *Basic steps in risk assessment*
   1. There are four basic steps in risk assessment, namely:
      a. *Hazard identification*: characterization of innate adverse toxic effects of agents.
      b. *Exposure assessment*: measurement or estimation of the intensity, frequency, and duration of human exposures to agents.
      c. *Dose-response assessment*: characterization of the relation between doses and incidences of adverse effects in exposed populations.
      d. *Risk characterization*: estimation of the incidence of health effects under the various conditions of human exposure.
   2. Risk characterization depends totally on the first three steps of risk process.

H. Hazard identification and dose-response assessment
   1. In this initial step, the potential for a xenobiotic to induce any type of toxic hazard is evaluated.
   2. Information is gathered and analyzed in a weight-of-evidence approach.
   3. The types of data usually consist of:
      a. Human epidemiology data.
      b. Animal bioassay data.
      c. Supporting data.
   4. Based on these results, one or more toxic hazards may be identified
      a. Cancer.
      b. Birth defects.
      c. Chronic toxicity.
      d. Neurotoxicity.
   5. *Illustration*: Steps in cancer risk assessment involve:
      a. Qualitative evaluation of all epidemiology studies, animal bioassay data, and biological activity (e.g., mutagenicity).
         1. The substance is classified as to carcinogenic risk to humans based on the weight of evidence.

2. If the evidence is sufficient, the substance may be classified as a definite, probable, or possible human carcinogen.

b. Quantify the risk for those substances classified as definite or probable human carcinogens.

I. Cancer classification schemes

1. The two primary cancer classification schemes are:
   a. Environmental Protection Agency (EPA).
   b. International Agency for Research on Cancer (IARC).
      1. The EPA and IARC classification systems are quite similar.
      2. The EPA's cancer assessment procedures have been used by several federal and state agencies. For example, the Agency for Toxic Substances and Disease Registry (ATSDR) relies on the EPA's carcinogen assessments.
2. The EPA's cancer assessment procedures uses several categories:
   a. The basis for sufficient human evidence is an epidemiology study that clearly demonstrates a causal relationship between exposure to the substance and cancer in humans.
   b. The data are determined to be limited evidence in humans if there are alternative explanations for the observed effect.
   c. The data are considered to be inadequate evidence in humans if no satisfactory epidemiology studies exist.
3. An increase in cancer in more than one species or strain of laboratory animals or in more than one experiment is considered sufficient evidence in animals.
4. Data from a single experiment can also be considered sufficient animal evidence if there is a high incidence or unusual type of tumor induced.
5. Normally, however, a carcinogenic response in only one species, strain, or study, is considered as only limited evidence in animals.

J. *Cancer slope*: The key risk assessment parameter derived from the EPA carcinogen risk assessment is the cancer slope factor.

1. This is a toxicity value that quantitatively defines the relationship between dose and response.

2. The cancer slope factor is a plausible upper-bound estimate of the probability that an individual will develop cancer if exposed to a chemical for a lifetime of 70 years.
3. The cancer slope factor is expressed as mg/kg/day.

K. The last step in risk assessment is to express the risk in terms of allowable exposure to a contaminated source.

L. Risk is expressed in terms of the concentration of the substance in the environment where human contact occurs. For example, the unit risk in air is risk per mg/m^3, whereas the unit risk in drinking water is risk per mg/L.

M. For carcinogens, the media risk estimates are calculated by dividing cancer slope factors by 70 kg (average weight of man) and multiplying by 20 m^3/day (average inhalation rate of an adult) or 2 L/day (average water consumption rate of an adult).

N. Exposure assessment involves exposed populations (general public or selected groups), types of substances (pharmaceuticals, occupational chemicals, or environmental pollutants), duration of exposure of a single substance or a mixture of substances (brief, intermittent, or protracted), and pathways and media (ingestion, inhalation, and dermal exposure).
1. Exposure assessment is a key phase in the risk assessment process because without an exposure, even the most toxic chemical does not present a threat.
2. All potential exposure pathways are carefully considered.
3. Contaminant releases, their movement and fate in the environment, and the exposed populations are analyzed.

O. All possible types of exposure are considered in order to assess the toxicity and risk that might occur due to these variables:
1. Physical environment.
2. Potentially exposed populations.

P. The physical environment may include considerations of:
1. Climate.
2. Vegetation.
3. Soil type.

   4. Groundwater.
   5. Surface water.

Q. Populations that may be exposed as the result of chemicals that migrate from the site of pollution are also considered.

R. Pollutants may:
   1. Be transported away from the source.
   2. Be physically, chemically, or biologically transformed.
   3. Accumulate in various media.

S. *Exposure pathways* may include:
   1. Groundwater.
   2. Surface water.
   3. Air.
   4. Soil.
   5. Food.
   6. Breast milk.

T. Because actual measurements of exposures are often not available, exposure models may be used. For example, in air quality studies, chemical emission and air dispersion models are used to predict the air concentrations to downwind residents.

U. *Risk characterization*: The final stage in the risk assessment process involves prediction of the frequency and severity of effects in exposed populations.
   1. Conclusions reached concerning hazard identification and exposure assessment are integrated to yield probabilities of effects likely to occur in humans exposed under similar conditions.
   2. Because most risk assessments include major uncertainties, it is important that biological and statistical uncertainties are described in the risk characterization.
   3. The assessment should identify which components of the risk assessment process involve the greatest degree of uncertainty.
   4. In some complex risk assessments, such as for hazardous waste sites, the risk characterization must consider multiple chemical exposures and multiple exposure pathways.

5. Simultaneous exposures to several chemicals, each at a subthreshold level, can often cause adverse effects by simple summation of injuries.
6. The assumption of dose additivity is most acceptable when substances induce the same toxic effect by the same mechanism.
7. When available, information on mechanisms of action and chemical interactions are considered and are useful in deriving more scientific risk assessments.
8. Individuals are often exposed to substances by more than one exposure pathway (e.g., drinking contaminated water, inhaling contaminated dust).
9. The total exposure will usually equal the sum of the exposures by all pathways.
10. *Higher exposure*: (a) living near an industrial complex, (b) living under a flight route, or (c) a child eating soil.
11. *More vulnerable*: (a) children, (b) pregnant women, (c) the elderly, and (d) Chronic Obstructive Pulmonary Disease (COPD) patients.

III. Major Sources of Environmental Hazards (Air Pollution, Water Pollution, Solid Waste, Contaminated Food, Environmental Factors, Weaponized Pathogens, Global Warming) and Their Health Impacts

A. *Outdoor air pollutants*: Major outdoor pollutants are (a) particulate matter (PM), (b) ozone, (c) nitrogen oxide, (d) carbon monoxide, and (e) sulfur dioxide.

1. Power plants, factories, and vehicles spew out harmful gases and small particles that can penetrate deep into human lungs, causing health problems.
   a. In strong sunlight, oxides of nitrogen from vehicle exhaust fumes form ozone at ground level, which can trigger asthma attacks.
   b. Heavy metals and persistent organic pollutants are carried by winds, contaminating water, and soil far from their origin.

   c. Industrial growth and rapid urbanization aggravate the problem, with the pressure felt most acutely in the mega-cities of the developing world.
   d. Use of cleaner fuels and technologies, refined motor engines, and public transportation are crucial in ensuring that children breathe clean air.
2. *Scope of outdoor air pollution*: Worldwide, outdoor air pollution contributes to:
   a. Estimated 800,000 deaths per year.
   b. Estimated 4.6 million healthy life-years lost per year.
   c. 65% deaths and lost life-years in Asia alone.
3. *Sources of outdoor air pollution*: May be quite different in rural and urban settings.
   a. Combustion of fossil fuels.
      1. Domestic heating.
      2. Power generation.
      3. Motor vehicles.
   b. Industrial processes.
      1. Cotton.
      2. Rug-making.
   c. Waste incineration.
   d. Natural processes.
      1. Thunderstorms.
      2. Volcanoes.
4. *Factors influencing outdoor air pollution*
   a. Climate: temperature, prevailing winds, and seasonal changes.
   b. Topography: hills and valleys and dominant vegetation.
   c. Cities.
   d. Surfaces.
5. *Particulate matter* refers to a complex heterogeneous mixture of solid and liquid.

a. *Sources*: (a) power plants and industry; (b) motor vehicles—domestic, coal burning; (c) natural sources (volcanoes, dust storms); and (d) small particles that form a surface for acid aerosol formation.
b. Primary particles originating from combustion sources usually consist of a carbonaceous core with chemicals (such as sulfates, metals, and polycyclic aromatic hydrocarbons) adsorbed to their surfaces.
c. In addition, secondary particles are formed by chemical reactions in the atmosphere of primary particles with gases (such as nitric oxides, ozone, and sulfur oxides, which are strong oxidants), leading to formation of nitrates and ammonia.
d. The specific composition and size distribution of PM varies by:
    1. Region.
    2. Time of year.
    3. Time of day.
    4. Weather conditions.

6. Particulate matter and route of entry and deposition in human organs:
    a. Coarse particles (2.5–10 μg) deposited in the upper respiratory tract and large airways.
    b. Fine particles (< 2.5 microns) may reach terminal bronchioles and alveoli.
    c. Particle size is the most important factor in determining where particles are deposited in the lung.
    d. Compared with large particles, fine particles can remain suspended in the atmosphere for longer periods and be transported over longer distances.
    e. Some studies suggest that fine particles have stronger respiratory effects in children than large particles.

7. *Health effects of PM*: Deposition of fine particles in distal airways may cause:
    a. Acute respiratory morbidity (pneumonia, asthma).
    b. Increased mortality (from all causes).
    c. Decreased lung function in children.

B. *Indoor air pollutants*
1. *Sources*: Indoor air quality is influenced by: (a) concentrations of outdoor air pollutants, (b) indoor sources of pollution, and (c) characteristics of the building and the habits of the residents.
2. Indoor air pollution may arise from the use of open fires; unsafe fuels; or the combustion of biomass fuels, coal, and kerosene.
3. Gas stoves or badly installed wood-burning units with poor ventilation and maintenance can increase the indoor levels of carbon monoxide, nitrogen dioxide, and particles.
    a. Other pollutants not associated with fuel combustion include building materials such as asbestos and cement, wood preservatives, and others.
    b. Volatile organic compounds may be released by various sources, including paints, glues, resins, polishing materials, perfumes, spray propellants, and cleaning agents.
    c. Formaldehyde is a component of some household products and can irritate the eyes, nose, and airways.

Table 5-4 Major Sources of Indoor Air Pollution

- Coal and biomass fuel can cause lung injury due to the inhalation of the ash particles.
- Suspended particulate matter increases the risk of acute respiratory infections.
- Carbon monoxide and other toxic gases may impair development and health.
- Secondhand tobacco smoke is a major concern.

4. *Note*:
   a. The indoor environment also reflects outdoor air quality and pollution.
   b. Outdoor pollution primarily results from the combustion of fossil fuels by industrial plants and vehicles.
   c. This releases carbon monoxide, sulfur dioxide, particulate matter, nitrogen oxides, hydrocarbons, and other pollutants.
   d. The characteristics of emissions and solid-waste disposal may vary for each specific industry (e.g., smelting, paper production, refining, and others).

Table 5-5 Sources and Products of Combustion

Sources	Products
Gas stoves and appliances	Carbon monoxide
Wood and coal stoves	Nitrogen dioxide
Gas and propane engines	Sulfur dioxide
Fireplaces	Nitrogenated compounds
Tobacco smoke	Particulate matter
Candles and incense	
Mosquito coils	

5. Chronic health conditions associated with indoor air pollutants.
   a. Decreased lung growth.
   b. Impaired pulmonary function.
   c. Increased susceptibility to chronic obstructive lung diseases, including asthma.

Table 5-6 Acute Health Consequences of Indoor Air Pollutants

- Coughing, wheezing, chest tightness
- Irritation of the mucous membranes (eyes, nose, throat)
- Increased airway responsiveness to allergens
- Increased incidence of acute respiratory illness
- Pneumonia
- Otitis media
- Tracheobronchitis
- Exacerbation of asthma

C. *Solid fuels*
   1. Solid fuels comprise only 10% to 15% of fuel used.
   2. Nearly one-half of the world's population uses solid fuels for cooking and heating homes.
   3. Two billion people are exposed to PM and gases at levels up to 100 times higher than in ambient air.
   4. Women and children are most exposed; levels may be 10 to 100 times above safety standards for ambient air.
   5. Biomass (wood, agricultural produce, straw, and dung) produces a wide variety of liquids, suspended particles, gases, and mixtures.
   6. *Coal: Products and health impact*
      a. Benzene, formaldehyde, sulfur, heavy metals, and fluoride.
      b. Affect the most vulnerable populations: women of child-bearing age, infants, and children in the poorest circumstances.

D. *Carbon monoxide: Composition and physiochemical properties*
   1. CO is a colorless, odorless gas formed by incomplete burning of carbon-based fuels.

2. CO's affinity for hemoglobin (Hb) is 240 to 270 times greater than that of oxygen.
   a. Decreases the capacity of Hb for carrying oxygen.
   b. Fetal Hb has a higher affinity for CO.
   c. CO causes a leftward shift of the oxyhemoglobin dissociation curve.
   d. Decreases oxygen delivery to tissues.
   e. Intoxication results in tissue hypoxia.
3. *Sources of carbon monoxide*
   a. Gas, kerosene, wood stoves, and coal: Incomplete oxidation during combustion in gas ranges and unvented gas or kerosene heaters may cause high concentrations of CO in indoor air.
   b. Worn or poorly adjusted and maintained combustion devices (e.g., boilers and furnaces) can be significant sources, especially if the fuel is of an unsuitable size, or if the system is blocked or leaking, such as chimneys and vents.
   c. Car, truck, or bus exhaust from attached garages, nearby roads, or parking areas can also be a source.
   d. CO is one of the components of tobacco smoke.

Table 5-7 Ways to Prevent CO Poisoning

- Keep fuel-burning appliances in good working condition.
- Check heating systems, chimneys, and vents regularly.
- Never burn charcoal indoors.
- Never leave a car running in a garage.
- Install CO detectors.

E. *Secondhand smoke*
   1. Sources and composition of secondhand smoke
      a. Smoke released from cigarettes, cigars, and pipes is composed of more than 3,800 different substances.
      b. Airborne particulate matter is 2 to 3 times higher in homes of smokers.
   2. Health impact of secondhand smoke
      a. Respiratory tract illness.
      b. Asthma.
      c. Middle ear effusions.
      d. Prenatal complications and low birth weight.
      e. Fire-related injuries.
      f. Sudden infant death syndrome (SIDS).
      g. Cancer.

F. *Solvents and volatile organic chemicals*
   1. *Composition*: Organic chemicals are widely used as ingredients in household products including paints, varnishes, wax, cosmetics, degreasing agents, wood preservatives, aerosol sprays, cleansers, disinfectants, moth repellents, air fresheners, and hobby products (e.g., alkanes, aromatic hydrocarbons, alcohols, aldehydes, ketones).
   2. *Sources*
      a. Solvents, fabric softeners, deodorizers, and cleaning products.
      b. Paints, glues, resins, waxes, and polishing materials.
      c. Spray propellants, dry cleaning fluids.
      d. Pens and markers.
      e. Binders and plasticizers.
      f. Cosmetics, hair sprays, and perfumes.
      g. Organic chemicals.
         1. All of these products can release organic compounds while they are being used, and, to some degree, when they are stored.

2. The average levels of several organic compounds in indoor air are 2 to 5 times higher than in outdoor air.
3. During certain activities, such as paint stripping, and for several hours immediately afterward, levels may be 1,000 times higher than outdoor levels.

3. Health impact of volatile organic chemicals (VOCs)
   a. VOCs vary greatly in their health effects: some are highly toxic, whereas some have no known effects on health.
   b. As with other pollutants, the extent and nature of the effects on health will depend on many factors including: level of exposure and duration of exposure.
4. *Acute* health impacts of volatile organic compounds
   a. Irritation of eyes and respiratory tract.
   b. Headache, dizziness, loss of coordination, nausea, visual disorders.
   c. Allergic reactions, including asthma and rhinitis.
5. *Chronic* health impacts of volatile organic compounds
   a. Damage to liver, kidney, blood system, and CNS.
   b. Cancer in humans.

G. Biologic pollutants
1. Animal dander, dust mites, molds, infectious agents, pollen.
2. Sources
   a. Humidifiers and stagnant water.
   b. Water-damaged surfaces and materials.
   c. Water vapor from cooking and showering.
   d. Air conditioning systems.
   e. Mattresses, upholstered furniture, and carpets.
3. Dust mites, fungi, and bacteria require moisture to proliferate.
4. Permeation of rain or groundwater into a building and condensation on cold interior surfaces can promote proliferation of microbes.

5. Water vapor is produced by people and pets, cooking, and showering and requires sufficient air exchange to prevent moisture problems.
6. Mattresses, upholstered furniture, and carpets are reservoirs for dust mites.
7. Molds have been associated with two types of effects: (a) allergic reactions and (b) toxic effects. Toxic effects may be caused by inhalation of mycotoxins.
8. Mold
   a. Source: Occurs in damp indoor spaces.
   b. *Manifestations*: More common among individuals with atopic disease.
   c. Allergies and nonspecific symptoms are common, but infections are rare.
   d. Mold-related diseases:
      1. Irritation of the airways and conjunctiva: eye irritation, cough, and sore throat.
      2. Headache.
      3. Difficulty in concentrating.
      4. Hypersensitivity reactions.
         a. Asthma.
         b. Allergic rhinitis.
      5. Infections.
         a. Thrush (candidiasis).
         b. Systemic infections (immunosuppression).
      6. Acute toxicity: Linked to pulmonary hemorrhage in infants.
   e. Hypersensitivity to molds is immediate (type 1) and includes acute asthma, allergic rhinitis, and urticaria.
   f. Colonization associated with chronic asthma is rare and serious and includes allergic bronchopulmonary mycosis and allergic mycotic sinusitis.

   g. Deep fungal infections are uncommon; serious, life-threatening diseases are not caused by common household molds.
      1. The major exception is aspergillosis.
   h. Molds usually infect devitalized tissue or an immunocompromised host.

H. *Sick building syndrome* (SBS) is assessed as follows:
   1. Discomfort is not related to specific illness.
   2. Effects appear to be linked to time spent inside the building.
   3. Cause of symptoms is unknown.
   4. Most complaints relieved soon after leaving the building (agent).
   5. *Manifestations*: Symptoms of identified illness attributed to airborne contaminants in the building.
   6. Etiology
      a. Inadequate building design.
      b. Occupant activities.
      c. Remodeled buildings operating in a manner inconsistent with their original design.
      d. Inadequate ventilation.
      e. Inadequate maintenance.
      f. Chemical and biological contaminants.
   7. Health impacts
      a. Headache.
      b. Irritations of eyes, nose, or throat.
      c. Dry cough.
      d. Dry or itchy skin.
      e. Difficulty in concentrating.
      f. Fatigue.
      g. Sensitivity to odors.

I. Radon gas
   1. Composition
      a. Radon is a radioactive gas released from soil and rocks.
      b. Geology of the area can predict levels in soil and water.

c. Radon concentrations indoors depend on construction site and building materials.
d. Radon is produced from the natural breakdown of thorium and uranium found in most rocks and soils. As it further breaks down, radon emits atomic particles.
e. Radon is the second leading cause of lung cancer.

2. Source and mechanism of disease causation
   a. Highest levels occur in basements and on the ground floor.
   b. Radon is a radioactive gas that comes from the soil.
   c. These particles are in the air we breathe and can be deposited in the lungs.
   d. The energy associated with these particles can alter DNA, leading to an increased risk of lung cancer.
   e. Radon can enter a new house through cracks or pores in concrete flooring and walls or through openings in the foundation, floor–wall joints, or loose pipes.
3. Health impacts
   a. Exposure to radon gas is the second-leading cause of lung cancer (after smoking) in the United States.
   b. About 14,000 people die each year from radon-related lung cancer.

J. Ozone (O_3)
   1. Structure, composition, and characteristics
      a. It is formed by a photochemical reaction of volatile organic compounds, $NO_2 + O_2$.
      b. It peaks in late afternoon.
      c. It is at its maximum level in hot, stagnant air.
      d. High concentrations increase asthma attacks in children.
      e. It is an important pollutant in many parts of the industrialized world.
      f. It is rarely measured in developing countries, so there is less information about its role in those countries.

g. It is a naturally occurring form of oxygen that provides a protective layer shielding the Earth from harmful ultraviolet radiation.
h. It also occurs in the lower atmosphere.
i. It is the major component of urban smog and a potent respiratory irritant that can also synergistically enhance a child's reaction to other air pollutants and pollen.
j. It is a secondary air pollutant formed in the atmosphere from a chemical reaction between hydrocarbons and nitrogen oxides in the presence of heat and sunlight.
    1. Ozone is a molecule composed of three atoms of oxygen.
    2. The third oxygen atom can detach from the ozone molecule and reattach to molecules of other substances, thereby altering their chemical composition.

2. Source: Scientific evidence shows that at concentrations that do not exceed public health standards, ozone has little potential to remove indoor air contaminants; there is no approval for its use in occupied spaces.

Table 5-8 The Health Effect of Ozone

- When inhaled, ozone can damage the lungs.
- Relatively small amounts can cause chest pain, coughing, shortness of breath, and throat irritation.
- Ozone may also exacerbate chronic respiratory diseases such as asthma and compromise the ability of the body to fight respiratory infections.

Source: www.epa.gov/iaq/pubs/ozonegen.html.

K. *Chromium: Health impacts*
1. Acute poisoning
    a. By ingestion: nausea, vomiting, hematemesis, acute renal failure.

b. By inhalation: acute pneumonitis, runny nose, sneezing, nosebleeds.
c. By skin contact: irritation, contact dermatitis, eczema.
d. Allergies, which are the most common health effect of chromium, including (1) contact dermatitis and (2) eczema.

2. Reproductive toxicity
   a. Low birth weight.
   b. Birth defects.
   c. Disturbed spermatogenesis.
3. Cancer
   a. Chromium is a human carcinogen and has been implicated in lung cancer.

L. *Cadmium*

1. Structure and composition
   a. Pure cadmium ores are relatively rare; they are mostly contained in zinc and lead ores.
   b. Cadmium is widely used in industry: electroplating, production of steel, plastics, batteries, fertilizers, pigments, ceramics and textiles.
2. Sources
   a. *Inhalation*
      1. Smoking and environmental tobacco smoke.
      2. Industrial emission as in waste incineration.
   b. *Ingestion* (main route of exposure)
      1. Food (internal organs of animals such as kidneys, tins of sardines, etc.).
      2. Elevated levels in drinking water (impurities in the zinc of galvanized pipes, solders, and metal fittings).
3. Health impacts
   a. *Acute toxicity*
      1. Inhalation: acute pneumonia.
      2. Ingestion: nausea, vomiting, abdominal cramps, diarrhea, liver and/or kidney lesions.

b. *Chronic toxicity*
   1. Inhalation: implicated as a carcinogen in lung and prostate cancer.
   2. Ingestion: based on lesions of the tubular function of the kidney.
   3. Proteinuria (β_2-microglobulin).
   4. Decreased reabsorption of calcium and phosphorus leading to osteoporosis and osteomalacia, thus predisposing to bone and hip fractures.
   5. Hypertension.
   6. Impairment in B cell immune response.

M. *Pesticides: Health impacts*
1. A number of epidemiological studies have found a significant association between cancer and domestic exposure to pesticides.
2. Evidence is increasing, but still limited because of the methodological weaknesses of the research (e.g., retrospective and case-control designs that are weak in direct determination of risk).
3. The following malignancies have been associated with exposure to pesticides:
   a. Brain tumor.
   b. Acute lymphocytic leukemia.
   c. Prostate cancer.
   d. Non-Hodgkin lymphoma.

N. *Lead: Health impact*
1. High blood lead level results in impaired intellectual ability in children.
2. High affinity for nerve tissue and hence neurotoxicity—hyperirritability, impaired memory, convulsions, coma, and death at high levels.
3. Interference with blood cells formation leading to anemia, as well as renal failure.

REVIEW QUESTIONS (MULTIPLE CHOICE)

Directions: Each of the following questions contains multiple suggested responses. Select the *one best* response to each question.

1. The therapeutic effect of Isotretinoin (Accutane) in treating acne has been documented. Accutane is a Vitamin A derivative, and large doses of Vitamin A are also known to be teratogenic. Which of the following statement(s) support(s) the role of Accutane as a teratogen?

a. Of women using Accutane during pregnancy, 20% have given birth to a defective child
b. Accutane received FDA approval with the stipulation that it is contraindicated during pregnancy
c. Both of the above
d. Neither of the above

2. Transport is the dominant source of air pollution in urban areas, with a large part of the urban population still being exposed to excesses of ambient quality levels for one or more pollutants. Which of the following is a known source of air pollution associated with transport?

a. Particulate matter
b. Nitrogen dioxide
c. Benzene
d. Ozone
e. All of the above

3. Long-term, low-level exposure to an electromagnetic field may cause adverse health effects via "chronic" impacts, or otherwise influence people's well-being. Scientific knowledge about the health effects of an electromagnetic field (EMF) is substantial and is based on a large number of epidemiological, animal, and in vitro studies. Many health outcomes have been examined. Which of the following health outcomes has been consistently linked with EMF?

a. Reproductive defects
b. Cardiovascular
c. Neuro-degenerative diseases
d. Childhood leukemia
e. None of the above

4. Toxic substances are often described by their abilities to cause adverse or unwanted health effects. Which of the following statements describes risk?

a. It is the capacity of a substance to cause an adverse effect in a specific organ or organ system
b. It reflects the probability that a hazard will occur under specific exposure conditions
c. It involves weighing of policy alternatives and selection of the most appropriate regulatory actions
d. It results in a statistically derived probability that an adverse effect will occur at a defined exposure level
e. None of the above

5. In the risk assessment process, the hazard identification step performs which of the following functions?

a. Characterizes the relationship between doses and incidences of adverse effects in exposed populations
b. Measures or estimates the intensity, frequency, and duration of human exposures to agents
c. Characterizes the innate adverse toxic effects of agents
d. Is the first step in the risk assessment process
e. None of the above

6. What data are most desirable to identify the primary hazard in the hazard identification step?

- **a.** Animal bioassay data
- **b.** Supporting data from cell and biochemical studies
- **c.** Human epidemiology data
- **d.** All of the above
- **e.** None of the above

7. The structure-activity relationship (SAR) has value in risk assessments in that it:

- **a.** Can often be used to predict possible toxicity
- **b.** Is used to design cell studies of the chemical's metabolism
- **c.** Can identify damage to DNA by actual testing of its chemical activity and biochemical structure
- **d.** Can often be used to predict possible toxicity
- **e.** None of the above

8. The EPA classification of a substance as a "probable human carcinogen" requires that the substance meet which of the following criteria?

- **a.** Inadequate evidence of cancer in humans and sufficient evidence of cancer in animals
- **b.** Limited evidence of cancer in animals
- **c.** Sufficient human evidence for a causal association between exposure and cancer
- **d.** Inadequate evidence in humans
- **e.** None of the above

9. The primary toxic effect that determines the type of procedure to be used in conducting a risk assessment is:

a. Lethality in laboratory animals
b. Evidence that the chemical is noncarcinogenic
c. The ability of the chemical to cause eye irritation
d. Evidence that the chemical is carcinogenic
e. None of the above

10. Although pesticides are used specifically to kill pests, many of them have environmental impacts as well as toxic effects on humans. The environmental impact of their use includes resistance development, killing of beneficial species, and environmental contaminant. Which of the following is (are) the result(s) of unintended contamination by pesticides?

a. Direct killing of organisms exposed to chemicals
b. Indirect killing via depletion of food or habitat
c. Groundwater contamination
d. Indirect contamination via food chains
e. All of the above

11. The primary method used to predict movement of substances in environmental media is:

a. Actual measurements of air and water pollutants at various places in the environment
b. Use of exposure models
c. Tagging pollutants with radioactive tracers and measuring the radioactivity at various times and locations within the environmental media
d. Exposure models
e. None of the above

12. Exposure assessment is a key phase in the risk assessment process because without an exposure, even the most toxic chemical does not present a threat. Which of the following step(s) is (are) included in the exposure assessment?

a. Characterization of the exposure setting (e.g., point source)
b. Identification of exposure pathways (e.g., groundwater)
c. Quantification of the exposure (e.g., μg/L water)
d. All of the above
e. None of the above

13. The main factors in the exposure assessment are:

a. Exposed populations (general public or selected groups)
b. Types of substances (pharmaceuticals, occupational chemicals, or environmental pollutants)
c. Duration of exposure (brief, intermittent, or protracted)
d. Pathways and media (ingestion, inhalation, and dermal exposure)
e. All of the above

14. A major aspect of the exposure assessment is to:

a. Determine the amount of exposure that must be reduced in order to comply with the acceptable risk level
b. Identify the exposure pathways
c. Measure the amount of a substance that is metabolized in the body
d. All of the above
e. None of the above

15. If actual measurements of exposures are often not available, exposure models may be used. Which of the following are considered as exposure pathways?

a. Groundwater
b. Air
c. Food
d. Breast milk
e. All of the above

16. The process in which the dose-response assessment and exposure assessments are integrated to predict risk in specific populations is known as which of the following?

a. Risk management
b. Hazard identification
c. Risk characterization
d. Risk modification
e. Risk quantification

17. What does an increased cancer risk of 2.0×10^{-6} mean?

a. It is likely that 2 persons in 1 million will develop the specific type of cancer in their lifetime due to exposure to the chemical
b. The xenobiotic for which the cancer risk assessment was performed is likely to cause cancer in 200 persons on a yearly basis
c. It is probable that 2 million persons will develop cancer if they are continuously exposed to the chemical for life
d. a and c only
e. None of the above

18. Power plants, factories, and vehicles spew out harmful gases and small particles that can penetrate deep into human lungs, causing health problems. In strong sunlight, oxides of nitrogen from vehicle exhaust fumes form ozone at ground level, which can trigger asthma attacks. Which of the following constitute major outdoor pollutants that can have an adverse effect on human health?

a. Particulate matter
b. Ozone
c. Carbon monoxide
d. a and c only
e. All of the above

19. Parental smoking and indoor and outdoor air pollutants have been associated with childhood asthma, and asthma is one of the leading causes of chronic disease among children. Which of the following is (are) indicative of increase in asthma severity among children with the condition?

a. Frequency and intensity of asthma attack
b. Number of emergency room visits during the year
c. Occurrence of asthma attacks that require intubations
d. a and b only
e. All of the above

20. Health consequences of secondhand tobacco smoke have been persistently observed. There is biological plausibility of exposure to secondhand smoke causing adverse neuro-development effects in children whose parents smoke. Which of the following statement(s) is (are) adequate concerning health effects of secondhand smoke?

a. Gaseous components of secondhand tobacco smoke may adversely affect lung defenses with effects on cilia and macrophage functions
b. Secondhand tobacco smoke may increase the severity of acute respiratory illness by irritating and inflaming the lungs

c. Secondhand tobacco smoke may contribute to eustachian tube dysfunction through a decrease in mucocilliary clearance, an increase in adenoidal hyperplasia, and an increase in mucosal swelling
d. a and c only
e. All of the above

21. Particle size is the most important factor in determining where particles are deposited in the lung. Deposition of fine particles in distal airways may cause which of the following?

a. Acute respiratory morbidity (pneumonia, asthma)
b. Increased mortality (from all causes)
c. Decreased lung function in children
d. All of the above
e. None of the above

22. Several toxic substances affect air quality. Some express their effect on indoor air quality, others on outdoor air quality. Which of the following is a major source of indoor air pollution?

a. Coal and biomass fuel
b. Suspended particulate matter
c. Carbon monoxide and other toxic gases
d. Secondhand tobacco smoke
e. All of the above

23. Toxic substances associated with indoor air pollutants can cause acute health consequences. Which of the following acute condition(s) is (are) expected to be associated with indoor air pollutants?

a. Irritation of the mucous membranes
b. Increased airway responsiveness to allergens
c. Decreased incidence of acute respiratory illness
d. a and b only
e. All of the above

24. Toxic substances associated with indoor air pollutants can cause chronic health effects. Which of the following chronic condition(s) is (are) expected to be associated with long-term exposure to indoor air pollutants?

a. Decreased lung growth
b. Impairment of pulmonary function
c. Increased susceptibility to chronic obstructive lung diseases, including asthma
d. All of the above
e. None of the above

25. Carbon monoxide (CO) is implicated as a potent and lethal air pollutant. Which of the following is (are) considered as the *major* source(s) of CO?

a. Gas, kerosene, wood stoves, and coal
b. Fireplaces and furnaces
c. Tobacco smoke
d. Vehicle exhaust in closed garage
e. All of the above

26. The clinical features of CO poisoning are highly variable, and symptoms vary from mild to very severe. As an environmental health specialist for the county's health department, you are at a scene with individuals exposed to CO. Which of the following manifestations would you expect to observe?

a. Dizziness, fatigue, dyspnea
b. Vomiting
c. Irritability
d. Unconsciousness, coma
e. All of the above

27. CO intoxication or poisoning carries lethal consequences. What are the primary prevention modalities that may help reduce the poisoning and mortality associated with CO?

- **a.** Limiting exposure to known CO sources
- **b.** Proper installation, maintenance, and use of combustion appliances
- **c.** Both of the above
- **d.** Neither of the above

28. Cigarette smoking during pregnancy has been associated with congenital anomalies. Which of the following statements support the role of smoking during pregnancy and children's health?

- **a.** Children whose mothers smoke have more respiratory problems than children whose mothers do not smoke
- **b.** Pneumonia and hospitalization in the first year of life are more frequent in children whose mothers smoke
- **c.** Infant mortality is higher in children born to women who smoked during pregnancy than in children of nonsmokers
- **d.** Infants of mothers who smoke have a higher risk of sudden infant death syndrome (SIDS) than infants of mothers who do not smoke
- **e.** All of the above

29. Molds are biologic pollutants and are associated with many health issues in the U.S. population. Which of the following conditions may be described as mold related?

- **a.** Airway and conjunctival irritation
- **b.** Hypersensitivity reactions such as asthma and rhinitis
- **c.** Infections due to immunologic reactions or effects
- **d.** a and b only
- **e.** All of the above

30. Mycotoxins are elaborated by mold, are associated with human disease, and cause acute and chronic effects. Which of the following mold toxins is (are) described as hepatotoxins and carcinogenic?

a. Tricothecenes
b. Ochratoxins
c. Citrinin
d. Aflatoxins
e. All of the above

31. The Sick Building Syndrome has been associated with loss of productivity at workplaces due to frequent absences from work by employees. As an environmental public health specialist expected to increase work attendance and hence productivity to improve the overall life quality of your community, which of the following will you consider as possible solutions to reduce the incidence of sick building syndrome?

a. Removing the source of pollutant
b. Increasing ventilation
c. Cleaning and changing air filters
d. Education and communication
e. All of the above

32. Radon is a radioactive gas released from soil and rocks and is second only to cigarette smoke as a carcinogenic substance in lung cancer. The radon migration system includes which of the following?

a. Gas-permeable layer
b. Plastic sheeting
c. Sealing and caulking

d. Vent pipe
e. Junction box
f. All of the above

33. The effects of exposure are influenced by individual susceptibility, which depends on age, developmental stage, nutrition, and social support. Pollutants in the indoor environment are potentially more hazardous to children than adults because their lungs are still growing and maturing; younger children breathe more air than older children or adults, and they spend more time indoors. Which of the following approaches will you consider in reducing indoor air pollutions?

a. Eliminating or controlling the sources of pollution
b. Ventilation with outdoor air to dilute and remove pollutants
c. Air cleaning by air filters and ionizers to remove some airborne particles
d. a and b only
e. All of the above

34. An estimated 4,000 toxic substances have been isolated in cigarette smoke. Some of these substances are clearly termed toxic and others as carcinogens. Which of the following substances in cigarette smoke have been categorized as carcinogenic?

a. Benzo-*a*-pyrene
b. *N*-Nitrosodimethylamine
c. Cadmium
d. a and c only
e. All of the above

35. A number of epidemiological studies have found a significant association between cancer and domestic exposure to pesticides. Evidence is increasing but still limited because of the methodological weaknesses of the research. Considering pediatric and adult malignancies, which of the following malignancies is (are) associated with exposure to pesticides?

- **a.** Brain tumor
- **b.** Prostate cancer
- **c.** Non-Hodgkin lymphoma
- **d.** a and c only
- **e.** All of the above

36. Prenatal and postnatal effects of environmental tobacco smoke predispose to several health conditions. You are an environmental health educator in a high-risk environment for tobacco, and you are required to address the health consequences of tobacco smoke. Which of the following conditions will you consider in your address?

- **a.** Sudden infant death syndrome
- **b.** Asthma
- **c.** Ear infection
- **d.** a and b only
- **e.** All of the above

37. Occupational exposure to mercury is not uncommon. A survey conducted by the National Institute for Occupational Safety and Health (NIOSH) estimated that 70,000 American workers may be exposed to mercury vapors on the job. The result of this study is more likely to associate which of these professions with mercury exposure?

a. Laboratory technicians
b. Plumbers
c. Dentist and dental hygienists
d. Miners
e. All of the above

38. Dichlorodiphenyltrichloroethane (DDT) exposure has been related to the disruption of the endocrine and immune systems in humans. Reproductive or immune system disruption may be caused by which of the following pesticides?

a. 1,2-dibromo-3-chloropane (DBCP)
b. Malathion
c. Parathion
d. Carbofuran
e. All of the above

39. The average amount of whole-body radiation exposure for an individual in the United States from all sources is estimated to be approximately 3.6 mSV (360 mrem) a year, or 0.01 mSv (1 mrem) per day. Because humans and other mammals are more sensitive to ionizing radiation relative to lower animals, higher doses of ionizing radiation may cause which of the following health effects in humans?

a. Mutations
b. Birth defects
c. Leukemia
d. Infertility
e. All of the above

40. The rising level of atmospheric carbon dioxide is indicative of global warming, and its impacts include diminished crop yields, loss of biodiversity, rising sea levels, and environmental health problems. The rate of global warming is due in part to increasing use of coal, oil, and gas to power the world's factories and vehicles. The widespread destruction of natural vegetation, particularly deforestation, contributes substantially to CO_2 emissions. As an environmental health specialist, which of the following policies are important in reducing greenhouse gas emission, thus minimizing global warming?

a. Improving energy efficiency
b. Replacing fossil fuels with "soft energy path" technologies—switching to solar, wind, or wave power to generate electricity
c. Reversing forest loss
d. Reducing chloroflurocarbons
e. Taxing the use of fossils fuels
f. All of the above

41. There are several sources of water pollution with point sources and nonpoint sources as the two broad categories. The sources of water pollution include agriculture, construction activities, urban street runoff, and fallout of airborne pollutants. In underdeveloped countries, contamination of waterways with microbial pathogens from human body wastes remains a major public health problem. Which of the following pathogens is (are) associated with diarrheal illness caused by sewage-tainted drinking water?

a. Vibrio cholera
b. Shigella
c. Salmonella
d. E. Coli
e. Rotavirus
f. Girada Lamblia
g. All of the above

42. The Environmental Protection Agency estimates that the United States currently generates more than 300 million metric tons of industrial hazardous wastes annually. The mismanagement of these wastes can adversely affect human health and reduce the quality of life. Which of the following threats is (are) posed by careless disposal of these wastes?

- **a.** Skin irritation and acute poisoning through direct contact
- **b.** Fire and/or explosions
- **c.** Air pollution
- **d.** Surface water contamination
- **e.** Groundwater contamination
- **f.** All of the above

43. Polychlorinated biphenyls (PCBs) are primarily employed as cooling liquids in electrical transformers and capacitors. The U.S. Environmental Protection Agency estimates that 91% of all Americans have detectable levels of PCBs in their fatty tissues. Also, PCBs are associated with several health effects. Which of the following adverse effects is (are) linked to PCBs?

- **a.** Acne-like skin disorders
- **b.** Burning sensation in eyes, nose, and throat
- **c.** Hepatic dysfunction
- **d.** All of the above
- **e.** None of the above

44. Dioxin is chemically related to PCBs and other chlorinated hydrocarbons. All of the following are correct about this substance *except*:

- **a.** Dioxin produces chloracne in rabbits
- **b.** Adverse effects in humans include immune system dysfunction
- **c.** Fetal toxicity is observed in humans
- **d.** None of the above
- **e.** All of the above

45. Environmental agents such as cigarette smoke, radon gas, sunlight, heavy metals, X-rays, and chemical pesticides are known to be carcinogenic and are believed to be human carcinogens. The exact mechanisms by which these substances induce tumors are not fully understood, but are thought to involve multiple steps. Which of the following statements is (are) accurate concerning the steps in tumor induction?

- **a.** Initiation is the first step, and involves a change in the genetic material
- **b.** The second step involves a process by which the initiated cells are exposed to another group of agents, termed promoters
- **c.** Environmental carcinogens can bind to DNA nucleotides, thus forming DNA-carcinogenic adducts, leading to genetic damage and abnormal cellular proliferation
- **d.** All of the above
- **e.** None of the above

46. The growing recognition of the extent of lead contamination in U.S. housing prompted the federal government to take action in October 1995 and demand the disclosure of lead hazards in pre-1978 housing in any Real Estate transaction. The need for this action was due to the environmental health impact of lead associated with house paint. Which of the following adverse effects of lead has been reported in the U.S. among children?

- **a.** High affinity for nerve tissue and hence neurotoxicity
- **b.** High blood lead levels, which result in impaired intellectual ability in children
- **c.** Both of the above
- **d.** Neither of the above

ANNOTATED ANSWERS

1. The correct answer is **C** (teratogens).

2. The correct answer is **E** (transport pollutants).

3. The correct answer is **D** (EMF and childhood leukemia). In 2001, an expert scientific working group of the World Health Organization's International Agency for Research on Cancer (IARC) reviewed studies related to the carcinogenicity of static and extremely low frequency (ELF) electric and magnetic fields. Using the standard IARC classification that weighs human, animal, and laboratory evidence, ELF magnetic fields were classified as "possibly carcinogenic to humans" on the basis of epidemiological studies of childhood leukemia, which showed, on average, a twofold excess of leukemia associated with living near power lines. The IARC "strength of evidence" for this risk is halfway between the strongest categories ("a human carcinogen" or a "probable carcinogen") and the weakest ("insufficient evidence" and "probably not a carcinogen") in their five categories. It is possible that there are other explanations for the observed association between exposure to ELF and childhood leukemia, and the extent of the hazard, if true, appears to be small.

4. The correct answer is **D** (risk process).

5. The correct answer is **D** (risk process).

6. The correct answer is **C** (risk assessment). Human data are the most desirable to identify the primary hazard in the hazard identification step and are given highest priority because there may be species differences in toxic response.

7. The correct answer is **D** (risk assessment and structure-activity relationship).

8. The correct answer is **D** (possible human carcinogen). With sufficient evidence in animals (*positive test results in more than one species or study*), the substance can be considered as a possible human carcinogen. Inadequate evidence in humans means that no satisfactory epidemiology study exists.

9. The correct answer is **D** (toxic effect of substances and risk assessment). The primary toxic effect that determines the type of procedure to be used in conducting a risk assessment is evidence that the chemical is carcinogenic. The risk assessment for carcinogens is quite different from that of noncarcinogens. Carcinogenic effects are viewed as nonthreshold effects, and noncarcinogenic effects are considered to have dose thresholds.

10. The correct answer is **E** (environmental impact of pesticide use). Direct killing of organisms exposed to chemicals, indirect killing via depletion of food or habitat, groundwater contamination, and indirect contamination via food chains are all environmental impacts of pesticide use (Nadakavukaren, *Our Global Environment*, 1995, pp. 301–309).

11. The correct answer is **D** (environmental media prediction method). Because actual measurements of environmental chemical exposure are often unavailable, exposure models are used. Models can predict future movement into areas that are currently free from contamination.

12. The correct answer is **D** (exposure assessment).

13. The correct answer is **E** (exposure assessment).

14. The correct answer is **B** (exposure assessment). A major aspect of the exposure assessment is to identify the exposure pathways. Also, all potential exposure pathways are carefully considered as well as contaminant releases, movement, and fate in the environment and the exposed populations.

15. The correct answer is **E** (exposure pathways).

16. The correct answer is **C** (risk characterization). Risk characterization is the process by which the dose-response assessment and exposure assessments are integrated to predict risk to specific populations. It is the final stage in the risk assessment process and involves the prediction of the frequency and severity of effects in exposed populations.

17. The correct answer is **A** (cancer risk estimation). An increased cancer risk of 2.0×10^{-6} means that it is likely that 2 persons in 1 million will develop the specific type of cancer in their lifetime due to exposure to the chemical.

18. The correct answer is **E** (major outdoor air pollutants).

19. The correct answer is **E** (health effect of air pollutants).

20. The correct answer is **E** (health effects of secondhand tobacco smoke—air pollutant).

21. The correct answer is **D** (health effect of particulate matter).

22. The correct answer is **E** (sources of indoor air pollutants).

23. The correct answer is **D** (acute health consequences of indoor air pollutants).

24. The correct answer is **D** (chronic health effects of indoor air pollutants).

25. The correct answer is **E** (sources of carbon monoxide).

26. The correct answer is **E** (signs and symptoms of carbon monoxide poisoning).

27. The correct answer is **C** (primary prevention of CO poisoning).

28. The correct answer is **E** (secondhand smoking and children's health).

29. The correct answer is **E** (health effects of biologic pollutants).

30. The correct answer is **D** (aflatoxins and carcinogenicity).

31. The correct answer is **E** (Sick Building Syndrome).

32. The correct answer is **E** (radon migration system). www.epa.gov/iaq/radon/construc.html

33. The correct answer is **E** (indoor air quality). www.epa.gov/iedweb00/pubs/hpguide.html

34. The correct answer is **E** (carcinogens in tobacco smoke).

35. The correct answer is **E** (pesticides and human cancer).

36. The correct answer is **E** (environmental tobacco smoke and health consequences).

37. The correct answer is **E** (occupational exposure to mercury).

38. The correct answer is **E** (pesticides and immune and reproductive health effects) (Nadakavukaren, *Our Global Environment*, 1995, pp. 312–317).

39. The correct answer is **E** (ionizing radiation and human health) (Nadakavukaren, *Our Global Environment*, 1995, pp. 377–380).

40. The correct answer is **F** (control of global warming).

41. The correct answer is **G** (sewage-tainted drinking water and causative pathogens of diarrheal disease).

42. The correct answer is **F** (hazardous waste and environmental health).

43. The correct answer is **D** (toxic substances and health effect) (Nadakavukaren, *Our Global Environment*, 1995, pp. 241–243).

44. The correct answer is **D** (dioxin and health effect).

45. The correct answer is **D** (carcinogenesis). Initiation is the first step and involves a change in the genetic material. Environmental carcinogens can bind to DNA nucleotides, thus forming DNA-carcinogenic adducts, leading to genetic damage and abnormal cellular proliferation. The second step involves a process by which the initiated cells are exposed to another group of agents, termed promoters. Environmental agents play a role in carcinogenesis as initiators and promoters—and both (Nasca & Pastides, *Fundamentals of Cancer Epidemiology*, 2001. pp. 60–61, 68–69).

46. The correct answer is **C** (environmental health effect of lead).

Chapter 6

Management and Policy Sciences in Public Health

Larry Holmes, Jr., Doriel Ward, Gbadebo Ogungbade, and Joan Nwuli

OVERVIEW

Management and policy sciences (MAPS) encompass the core disciplines of public health and play a significant role in the policy development and assurance of public health services. MAPS is a multidisciplinary field of inquiry and practice concerned with the delivery, quality, and costs of health care for individuals and populations. This description of MAPS assumes both a managerial and a policy concern with the structure, process, and outcomes of health services, including the costs, financing, organization, outcomes, and accessibility of care.

This chapter presents the role of policy in public health services implementation and intervention designs to control diseases and promote health, the governmental role in health policy development, the substance of public health law, and the public health federal regulations, with an emphasis on the Health Insurance Portability and Accountability Act (HIPAA). Public health ethics is presented in contrast to medical ethics, focusing mainly on human subjects in research as well as the elements of informed consent. Equity in health is presented in terms of the inequality in the provision of quality care due to personal characteristics such as race/ethnicity, gender, socioeconomic status, and age, with stress on the health effects of insurance coverage and racial/ethnic disparities.

I. Management and Policy Sciences and Public Health

A. Policy development, organization, and management of public health services are essential functions of public health.

B. Policy development as a core function of public health involves:

1. Broad community involvement.
2. Promotion of the scientific basis of decision-making.
3. Strategic approach.
4. Development of comprehensive public health policies.

C. Policy development serves as a core function of public health. The implementation of public health services requires policy development and planning or management:

1. Systematic community-wide planning for health improvement.
2. Developing and tracking measurable objectives.
3. Developing policy and legislation to the practice of public health.
4. Implementing joint evaluation with medical care system.
5. Leadership development at all levels.

D. Framework for examining public health system performance

1. The framework for examining public health system performance involves capacity, process, and outcomes.
2. The capacity level refers to the inputs that involve interaction with workforce, information, organization, relationship, facilities, and funding.
3. The process that is the essential public health services refers to the core functions of public health: assessment, policy development, and assurance.
4. The outcome refers to the output (program and services consistent with mandates, community needs, and priorities) that leads to the outcomes (improved organizational performance and improved program performance).

II. General Notion of Policy Formulation and Implementation

A. If public health is to meet its substance of disease control and health promotion, it must rely on evidence-based policies.

B. The use of evidence-based policy and practice can effectively lead to improvement in the health of the population.
C. The movement for evidence-based policy and practice and for the use of research evidence in the work of the professions started in medicine in the early 1990s. It has grown in influence and spread across a number of other fields.
D. Building on a tradition of evidence-based medicine, this approach is receiving increasing attention in new fields of professional practice such as education, social work, criminal justice, regeneration, and others.
E. The process of sourcing the evidence must be incorporated as an integral part of the policy formulation itself.
F. The effectiveness of this approach is also based on the integrity of the processes of sourcing the evidence, interpreting the information, utilizing the knowledge, understanding and adopting the evidence, evaluating and adapting it, and applying and acting on it.
G. The overall process for the evidence-based policy formulation is illustrated by:
   1. The policy idea.
   2. Sourcing the evidence, implying knowledge, research, ideas/interest, politics, and economics.
   3. Evidence usage.
   4. Consideration of the capacity to implement.
H. *Stages in policy development*:
   1. Problem identification.
   2. Priority setting.
   3. Policy formulation and design.
   4. Passage of policy instruments.
   5. Implementation.
   6. Evaluation.
I. *Tools and resources to support policy development*:
   1. Data gathering and analysis.
   2. Research effectiveness of strategies.

3. Media strategies (in collaboration with the communications coordinator).
4. Training.
5. Evaluation.

III. Health Policies and the Governmental Role in Development and Implementation

A. Health policy involves all sectors of the government:
   1. *Federal*
      a. U.S. Department of Health and Human Services
         1. Agencies include the National Institutes for Health (NIH), the Centers for Disease Control and Prevention (CDC), The U.S. Food and Drug Administration (FDA), the Agency for Health Research Quality (AHRQ), etc.
         2. Programs include Medicare, Medicaid, State Children's Health Insurance Program (SCHIP), Maternal and Child Health (MCH), and family planning.
   2. *State*
      a. Departments of health, human services, or social services.
      b. Divisions of insurance.
      c. Medical schools and affiliated teaching hospitals.
   3. *Local*
      a. Departments of public health.

B. *Spending on health*:
   1. Accounts for a sizable share of state spending; half from federal funds.
   2. Total U.S. state health spending in the years 2002–2003 accounted for \$1.1 trillion.

C. *States' role in health policy*
   1. *Regulator*
      a. Health professional licensing.
      b. Health facilities licensing.
      c. Insurance companies and managed care organizations regulations.

2. *Purchaser*
    a. Medicaid beneficiaries.
    b. State Children's Health Insurance Program (SCHIP).
    c. State employees and retirees.
3. *State health spending is dominated by Medicaid*
    a. Medicaid is administered by the states with federal oversight and shared federal/state financing (57% federal).
    b. Medicaid provides health and long-term care services for more than 52 million low-income people.
        1. 39 million adults and children in low-income families.
        2. 13 million frail elders and people with disabilities, including more than 6 million Medicare beneficiaries.
4. Pays for nearly 1 in 5 healthcare dollars and 1 in 2 nursing home dollars.
5. Large variation across states in eligibility and scope of benefits.
6. *Provider*
    a. Facilities for the developmentally disabled and mental health hospitals.
    b. State-operated nursing homes and veterans' homes.
    c. Medical schools and affiliated teaching hospitals.
    d. Prisons:
        1. States spent $4.0 billion on inmate medical care in 2003.
        2. Increase in spending as a result of larger prison population, increase in HIV/AIDS, and aging of prison population.
    e. Public and population health.
    f. Programs for targeted populations.

D. *Public health functions of the state*
1. Vital statistics records and reporting.
2. Disease surveillance.
3. Injury prevention and public safety.
4. Staff and operate pathology lab.
5. Medical research.
6. Protection against environmental hazards.

E. *Specific services provided by the state* (*Source: Milbank Memorial Fund, The National Association of State Budget Officers, and the Reforming States Group, 2002–2003 State Health Expenditure Report, June 2005*)
   1. Title V.
   2. Maternal and Child Health Program.
   3. Drug assistance for seniors.
   4. Chronic disease hospitals and programs.
   5. Hearing aid assistance.
   6. Adult day care for persons with Alzheimer's disease.
   7. Health grants.
   8. Medically-handicapped children.
   9. Women, Infants, and Children (WIC) programs.
   10. Pregnancy outreach and counseling.
   11. Chronic renal disease treatment programs.
   12. AIDS treatment.
   13. Breast and cervical cancer screening and treatment.
   14. Tuberculosis (TB) programs.
   15. Emergency health services.
   16. Adult genetics programs.
   17. Phenylketonuria (PKU) testing.

F. *Congress and health policy*
   1. Congress plays a major role in development of health policy:
      a. Medicare.
      b. Medicaid.
      c. National Institutes of Health.
      d. Health policy is a bi-partisan priority.
      e. Authority spread across several committees.
      f. Involvement includes regulatory, programmatic, financing, and oversight.
   2. *Top three healthcare priorities for the U.S. Congress, 2005* (*Source:* KFF/Harvard School of Public Health, *Health Care Agenda for the New Congress*, conducted November 4–28, 2004)
      a. Lowering cost of health care and insurance—63%.

   b. Increasing number of Americans without insurance—57%.
   c. Improving nation's ability to respond to bioterrorism—50%.
3. *Congressional legislation on health care (illustrative legislations)*
   a. Enactment of Medicare and Medicaid (1965).
   b. Employee Retirement Income Security Act (1974).
   c. Americans with Disabilities Act (1990).
   d. Family Medical Leave Act (1993).
   e. Temporary Assistance for Needy Families (1996).
   f. Health Insurance Portability and Accountability Act (1996).
   g. State Children's Health Insurance Program (1997).
   h. Medicare Modernization Act (2003).
4. *Senate Health, Education, Labor and Pension (HELP) Committee*—chief health responsibilities:
   a. Aging policy.
   b. Biomedical research and development.
   c. Domestic activities of the American National Red Cross.
   d. Individuals with disabilities.
   e. Occupational safety and health, including the welfare of miners.
   f. Public health.
5. *House Committee on Energy and Commerce*—chief health responsibilities:
   a. Medicaid.
   b. Medicare.
   c. Public health programs.
   d. Food and drug safety.
   e. Hospital construction, mental health and research, biomedical programs, and health protection in general.
6. *House Committee on Ways and Means*—chief health responsibilities:
   a. Government payments for programs in Social Security Act: Medicare, welfare (TANF), Supplemental Security Income (SSI), Social Services (Title XX).

    b. Tax credits and related matters in the tax code dealing with health insurance premiums.
7. *House Committee on Finance*—chief health responsibilities:
    a. Health programs under the Social Security Act and health programs financed by a specific tax or trust fund, including: Medicaid, Medicare, SCHIP, welfare (TANF), Maternal and Child Health block grant, SSI, ERISA (with HELP Committee).
    b. Revenue measures generally, except as provided in the Congressional Budget Act of 1974.

IV. Public Health Laws and Application to Health Promotion and Disease Prevention

A. Constitutional right to privacy: *Whalen v. Roe* grants limited right to health information privacy
B. Privacy is inherent in U.S. history and the Constitution
    1. Federal law
        a. Privacy Act 1974.
        b. Health Insurance Portability and Accountability Act (HIPAA) privacy rules.
    2. State law
        a. Disease specific.
        b. Extra confidentiality for certain conditions.
    3. Tort
C. Public Law 104-191: Health Insurance Portability and Accountability Act of 1996
    1. Electronic transactions and code sets
        a. Standardizes the data content and format of 10 financial or administrative transactions related to health care (e.g., claims, payments).
        b. Standardizes medical codes (no local codes, e.g., "Y" codes).
    2. Privacy of Individually Identifiable Health Information (PIIHI)
        a. Regulates uses and disclosures of individually identifiable health information.

   b. Provides patient rights with respect to their health information.
   c. Establishes requirements to ensure privacy of patient.
3. HIPAA-covered entities
   a. *Health plans*
      1. Provides or pays for the cost of healthcare services.
      2. Includes Medicaid, Medicare, HealthChoice, Veterans Health Program, Military Health Plan, Indian Health Service, and others.
      3. Excludes most other government-funded programs.
   b. Healthcare providers who conduct any of the HIPAA-regulated transactions electronically.
   c. Healthcare clearinghouses (not applicable to Division of Public Health).

D. *Privacy regulation*
1. The privacy regulation establishes a federal floor of safeguards to protect the confidentiality of health information.
2. Applies to Protected Health Information (PHI), which is:
   a. Individually identifiable health information.
   b. Transmitted or maintained in any form or medium (electronic, written, oral).
3. PHI is any information, including demographic information, collected from an individual that:
   a. Is created or received by a healthcare provider, health plan, employer, or healthcare clearinghouse.
   b. Relates to the past, present, or future physical or mental health or condition of an individual; the provision of health care to an individual; or the past, present, or future payment of the provision of health care to an individual.

E. *HIPAA: Individual rights*
1. Right to be informed of protections on and use of their health information through a notice of privacy practices.
2. Right to inspect, copy, and review their record.

3. Right to request amendments to their record.
4. Right to request restrictions on use and disclosure of health information.
5. Right to request reasonable personal communications.
6. Right to an accounting of disclosures of their health information.
7. Right to file a complaint against covered entity.

V. Public Health Ethics

A. Ethical values include:
   1. Respect for persons or autonomy.
   2. Trusting relationships.
   3. Economic harms.

B. Medical ethics is primarily concerned with patient–provider relationships or interactions.

C. Public health ethics is concerned with institutions and populations.
   1. The foci of medical ethics are autonomy, goodness and beneficence.
   2. Public health ethics focuses on interdependence, participation, and scientific information.

D. Human subjects in research
   1. *Nuremberg Code* (*Human Experimentation*): The voluntary consent of the human subject is absolutely essential. This means that the person involved should have legal capacity to give consent; should be so situated as to be able to exercise free power of choice, without the intervention of any element of force, fraud, deceit, duress, over-reaching, or other ulterior form of constraint or coercion; and should have sufficient knowledge and comprehension of the elements of the subject matter involved as to enable him or her to make an informed and enlightened decision. This latter element requires that before the acceptance of an affirmative decision by the experimental subject, there should

be made known to him or her the nature, duration, and purpose of the experiment; the method and means by which it is to be conducted; all inconveniences and hazards to be reasonably expected; and the effects upon his or her health or person that may possibly come from his or her participation in the experiment.

2. The duty and responsibility for ascertaining the quality of the consent rests upon each individual who initiates, directs, or engages in the experiment. It is a personal duty and responsibility that may not be delegated to another with impunity.
3. Title 45 (Public Welfare Department of Health and Human Services), Part 46 (Protection of Human Subjects), of the *Code of Federal Regulations* (CFR) sets the guidelines for the protection of human subjects in research.
4. *Belmont Report on Human Subject Protection (National Commission for the Protection of Human Subjects of Biomedical and Behavioral Research)*: One of the charges to the Commission was to identify the basic ethical principles that should underlie the conduct of biomedical and behavioral research involving human subjects and to develop guidelines that should be followed to ensure that such research is conducted in accordance with those principles. In carrying out these principles, the Commission was directed to consider:
    a. The boundaries between biomedical and behavioral research and the accepted and routine practice of medicine.
    b. The role of assessment of risk-benefit criteria in the determination of the appropriateness of research involving human subjects.
    c. Appropriate guidelines for the selection of human subjects for participation in such research.
    d. The nature and definition of informed consent in various research settings.

5. *World Medical Association Declaration of Helsinki—Ethical Principles for Medical Research involving Human Subjects*
   a. The World Medical Association has developed the Declaration of Helsinki as a statement of ethical principles to provide guidance to physicians and other participants in medical research involving human subjects.
   b. Medical research involving human subjects includes research on identifiable human material or identifiable data.
   c. It is the duty of the physician to promote and safeguard the health of the people. The physician's knowledge and conscience are dedicated to the fulfillment of this duty.
   d. The Declaration of Geneva of the World Medical Association binds the physician with the words, "The health of my patient will be my first consideration," and the International Code of Medical Ethics declares that, "A physician shall act only in the patient's interest when providing medical care which might have the effect of weakening the physical and mental condition of the patient."

VI. Health Disparities: Insurance and Race/Ethnicity

A. Health insurance and population health
B. Most Americans have health insurance, but millions do not; many who are well covered today may find themselves uninsured or underinsured in the future.
C. Studies have persistently shown the nexus between disease prognosis and mortality and insurance coverage.
D. Without adequate insurance coverage, people simply do not get the care they need, when they need it.
E. There are differences between insured and uninsured regarding barriers to health care.

Table 6-1 Differences between Insured and Uninsured with Respect to Obstacles to Receiving Health Care

Obstacles to Health Care	Uninsured (%)	Insured (Public and Private) (%)
Postpone seeking care because of cost	47	15
Need care but did not get it	35	9
Did not fill a prescription because of cost	37	13
Had problems paying medical bills	36	16
Contacted by collection agency about medical bills	23	8

Source: Kaiser 2003 Health Insurance Survey

F. *Health risk—uninsured versus insured*
   1. Uninsured people, compared with those privately insured, are less likely to be diagnosed with early onset tumor (prostate, breast, melanoma, colorectal cancer) and are more likely to be diagnosed with late onset malignancy.
   2. People in poor health are twice as likely to have a lengthy spell without coverage.

G. *Insurance distribution*
   1. At age 65, most people in the United States qualify for Medicare.
   2. Before age 65, we rely on various sources of coverage.
   3. About 15% of the non-elderly are covered under public programs—mostly Medicaid, which is a safety net program for certain low-income people: children, parents of dependent children, pregnant women, and people with disabilities who cannot work.
   4. The vast majority of people under age 65 rely on private health insurance.

5. The $1.9 trillion healthcare system in 2004 indicated that more than one-third of total healthcare spending was financed by private health insurance.
6. More than 60% of the non-elderly get private health insurance at work, as a benefit from their own job or as the spouse or dependent of a working family member.
7. About 5% of the non-elderly buy health insurance on their own in what is called the "individual insurance market."
8. The rest—18% or almost 46 million non-elderly Americans—are uninsured.

H. *Private insurance model*
1. Indemnity.
2. "Managed care."
    a. Preferred provider organization (PPO).
    b. Health maintenance organization (HMO).
    c. Point of service (POS).
3. "Consumer-directed" health arrangements.
4. Most people with private insurance have some form of managed care, implying that coverage is most comprehensive when the physician is seen in a specified network. Care provided out of network may not be covered, or the policyholder may be required to pay more out of pocket. Different models vary in specifics of network policies, how they are financed, access to specialists, benefits, and cost-sharing.
5. Consumer directed health plans are characterized by high cost-sharing and represent a fundamental shift whereby the consumer is responsible for more of the purchasing of healthcare plans.

I. *Health insurance dynamics*
1. There are 45 million uninsured in a 1-year snapshot, but 80 million people may lack coverage for at least 1 month over a 2-year period.

2. Coverage options can change with:
   a. Loss or change of job.
   b. Change in family status (e.g., divorce, death of spouse).
   c. Birthday (e.g., 19th).
   d. Relocation—moving.
   e. Change in health status.
3. Similarly, the snapshot shows 5% in the individual market, but one in four adults will try to buy individual coverage during a 3-year period.
4. On average, 2 million Americans lose or change coverage every month.
5. Of these 2 million people, most will be uninsured for at least 30 days, then obtain new coverage. However, for some it will take a year or longer before they regain insurance.
6. Insurance eligibility.

J. *Employer-sponsored insurance* is less likely to be offered to:
   1. Employees of small relative to large firms.
   2. Part-time/seasonal workers compared to full-time.
   3. Low-wage workers.
   4. Newly hired workers (waiting periods).
   5. Dependents relative to employees.
   6. Retirees.

K. Eligibility is not based on health status.

L. *Individual insurance*
   1. Purchased by individuals.
   2. Age and health status are a determining factor (medical underwriting).

M. *Health conditions determining individual insurance*: Individual insurance may be denied due to the following health conditions:
   1. *Always denied*
      a. Cancer.
      b. Multiple sclerosis.

c. HIV/AIDS.
d. Pregnancy.
e. Diabetes.
f. Stroke.

2. *Often denied*
    a. Overweight.
    b. High blood pressure.
    c. Cancer history.
    d. Asthma.
3. *Sometimes denied*
    a. Acne.
    b. Hay fever.

N. *Expanding health insurance coverage*
1. *Expanding public coverage*
    a. Expansions of Medicaid/SCHIP at the state level.
    b. National health insurance program: "Medicare for All."
2. *Expanding private group coverage through current employer-sponsored system*
    a. Financial incentives for employers to provide coverage.
    b. Employer mandates.
    c. New group insurance options, especially for small employers.
3. *Subsidizing purchase of private health insurance through tax credits and deductions*
    a. Individual tax credits/deductions to subsidize insurance premiums.
    b. Increased utilization of health savings accounts (HSAs) for certain types of health insurance.

O. *Racial/ethnic disparities in health*
1. Health equity refers to providing care that does not vary in quality because of personal characteristics such as gender, age, ethnicity/race, geographic location, and socioeconomic status.

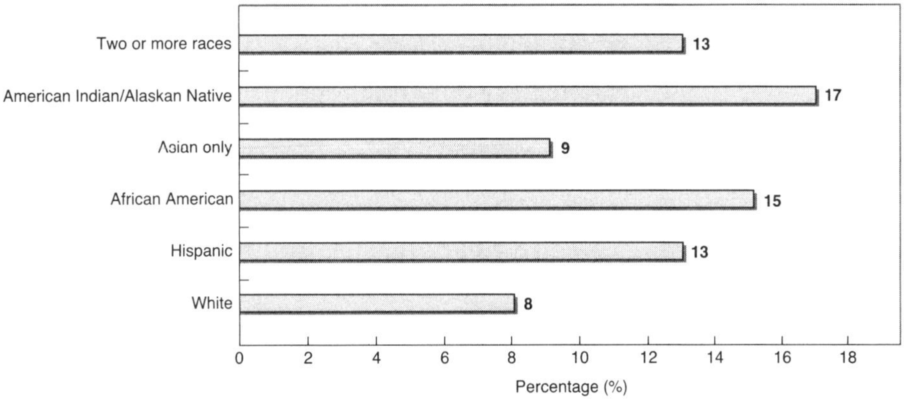

Figure 6-1 Percentage of Sample U.S. Residents with Fair or Poor Health by Race/Ethnicity, 2004

Table 6-2 Poverty Status* of US Residents, Age 65 and Younger, 2005

Race/Ethnicity	Non-poor (%)	Near Poor (%)	Poor (%)
White (*n* = 166.6 million)	74	14	12
Hispanic (*n* = 40.8 million)	42	29	29
African American (non-Hispanic) (*n* = 32.6 million)	46	21	33
Asians only (*n* = 11.8 million)	68	16	17
American Indian/Alaska Native (*n* = 1.5 million)	43	23	34
Two or more races (*n* = 4.2 million)	59	20	21

*The poverty status is based on the federal level (2005) of $19,971 for a family of four.

Source: Urban Institute and Kaiser Commission on Medicaid and the Uninsured, analysis of March 2006 Current Population Survey.

2. *U.S. population by race/ethnicity*: Whites make up the majority (67%), followed by Hispanics (14%), African Americans (non-Hispanic) (12%), Asian only (4%), two or more races (1%), American Indian/Alaskan Natives (0.7%), and Native Hawaiian/Pacific Islanders (0.1%).
3. African Americans and Hispanics, compared with Whites, are more likely to have uncontrolled diabetes and to present with short-term and long-term complications.
4. African Americans and Hispanics are more likely to be diagnosed with AIDS and to die from HIV infection, compared with Whites.
5. African Americans relative to Whites are less likely to experience increases in the quality of care.

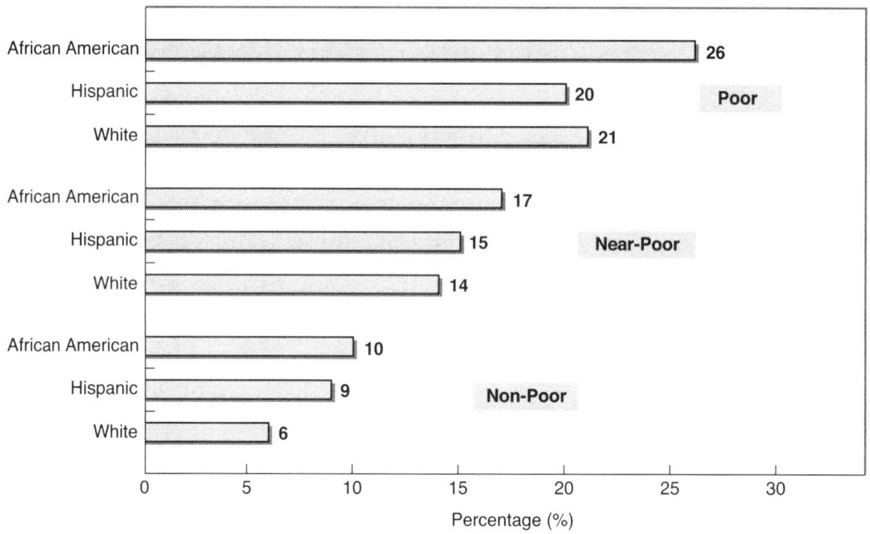

Figure 6-2 Sample of U.S. Residents with Fair or Poor Health by Race/Ethnicity and Poverty Status, 2004

VII. Public Health Services: Organization and Management Theories

A. *Systems Thinking and Systems Tools*

1. Concerns with understanding and guiding change in organizations, implying the examination of the overall structures, patterns, and cycles in systems, rather than focusing on isolated or specific events in the systems.
2. Understanding how system thinking and tools are used in organization requires an understanding of a system in the first place.
   a. A system is an organized collection of parts that are highly integrated to accomplish an overall goal.
   b. The system has various inputs, which go through certain processes to produce certain outputs, which together, accomplish the overall desired goal for the system.
3. In public health systems thinking reflects the potentials of public health administrators/mangers to identify solutions that address multiple problems within the system, hence maximizing improvement throughout the entire public health system (project or program).
4. Secondly, systems thinking implies long-term effect or solutions of an intervention and not short-term effect of public health intervention.
5. Systems thinking further utilizes a bigger picture in the intervention model of public health initiative to control disease and promote health.
   a. *Vignette:* If insect A causes cellulites and insect A feeds on insect B (a potent pathogen for acute bacterial meningitis), is systems thinking applied here by developing pesticides to eliminate insect A only?
   b. *Solutions:* The approach to eliminate insect A only by developing a potent pesticide is not a systems thinking tool because the elimination of insect A will lead to a

greater health problem, acute bacterial meningitis. Systems thinking will require an integrated pest management, thus eliminating all insects associated with human health.

6. Systems thinking claims that:
   a. Parts of systems communicate with each other
   b. Systems have an environment with communication entities
   c. Systems are continuously changing, with a small stimulus causing a large effect or no effect all (i.e., global warming)
   d. Systems behavior cannot be predicted from the behavior of its parts
   e. Systems as a whole works differently from its parts
   f. Parts, per se, cannot accomplish what systems are capable of accomplishing—parts cannot contain the whole
7. Organization is defined by complexity and the systems that create the complexity is adaptive, implying organizational change and unpredictability of the future.
8. Public health problems are complex because there are so many factors that determine the health of the population. In effect, public health issues cannot be subjected to a simple cause and effect model.
9. Systems thinking thus claims to identify the real problems by going beyond the cause and effect model, thus providing potential solutions.

B. *Chaos Theory*
   1. Chaos theory deals with unpredictable complex systems.
      a. This theory originates, in part, from the work of Edward Lorenz, a meteorologist, who simulated weather patterns on a computer.
   2. Rather than understanding a changing system as series of causal steps, chaos theory postulates a point in the system in the future, an attractor, which pulls the system toward it.

    a. When the system is unpredictable at a certain stage, the future may unfold quite differently, depending upon what little difference occurred

  3. In public health organization and management, the chaos theory reflects the complexity and unpredictability of public health services because of its relations with other systems (state, federal government, local government, private sectors etc.).

C. *Contingency Leadership Theory (CLT)*

  1. CLT was proposed by the Austrian psychologist Fred Fiedler
  2. It classifies leaders into: (a) those motivated by the need to accomplish assigned tasks, implying task-oriented, (b) those motivated by close and supportive relations with members of the group, hence people-orientated.
  3. The effectiveness of the leader is contingent upon:
    a. Leader's personality
    b. Characteristics of the leadership situation

D. *Douglas McGregor's XY Theory*

  1. Douglas McGregor, an American social psychologist, proposed the famous XY theory in the 1960s.
  2. McGregor's XY Theory remains central to organizational development, and to improving organizational culture.
  3. McGregor's XY theory is indicative of the natural rules for managing people, which under the pressure of day-to-day business are all too easily forgotten.
  4. This theory maintained that there are two fundamental approaches to managing people. (a) Many managers tend toward theory x, and generally get poor results. (b) Enlightened managers use theory y, which produces better performance and results, and allows people to grow and develop.

E. *Path-Goal Theory of Leadership (Robert House, 1971)*
   1. Developed to describe the way leaders encourage and support their followers in achieving the goals they have been set by making the path that they should take clear and easy.
   2. Maintains that leaders can affect the performance, motivation, and satisfaction of a group by: (a) offering rewards after achieving the performance goal, (b) clarifying paths towards these goals, and (c) removing obstacles or barriers to performance.
   3. This theory identifies four types of leadership styles:
      a. Directive
      b. Supportive
      c. Participative
      d. Achievement-oriented

REVIEW QUESTIONS (MULTIPLE CHOICE)

Directions: Each of the following questions contains multiple suggested responses. Select the *one best* response to each question.

1. Public health needs to help communities increase access to safe, nutritious food grown in a sustainable way so that people can make healthy food choices. Such public health efforts can contribute to the prevention and control of which of the following ailments or conditions?

- **a.** Obesity
- **b.** Diabetes
- **c.** Cancer
- **d.** Heart disease
- **e.** All of the above

2. Health policy is a multidimensional process. Which of the following statements is (are) correct regarding the role of Congress in U.S. health policy?

a. Congress plays an integral role in the development, financing, and oversight of public and private sector health policies
b. Congressional health policy agendas are driven by a range of forces, including the presidential budget, political agenda, lobbying, and advocacy
c. Both of the above
d. Neither of the above

3. More than 60% of non-elderly Americans get private health insurance at work as a benefit from their own job or as the spouse or dependent of a working family member. Data have consistently shown that having private insurance increases the risk for late diagnosis from melanoma, prostate, and breast cancer. Which of the following conditions may result in a change in insurance coverage?

a. Loss of job
b. Change in family status
c. Birthday
d. Change in health status
e. All of the above

4. Private insurance through an employer differs from individual insurance. Which of the following statements is (are) indicative of the basic distinction?

a. Eligibility is not based on health status in individual insurance
b. Eligibility is based on age and health status in employer-sponsored insurance
c. Both of the above
d. Neither of the above

5. Private health insurance coverage is not a right but a service for those who can afford it. All of the following are true regarding coverage *except*:

- **a.** Private insurance is a mainstay of health coverage for most Americans, but access, affordability, and adequacy of coverage are not guaranteed
- **b.** Despite limited access to coverage, disease prognosis is not related by any known study or body of research to insurance coverage
- **c.** Difficulty of getting/keeping private coverage increases with health problems, especially during coverage transitions
- **d.** Regulation to limit risk selection involves trade-offs: access versus adequacy versus affordability
- **e.** Additional public policy responses are needed to subsidize and expand coverage

6. The Healthy People 2010 objective indicates the need to eliminate health disparities. Which of the following strategies should be considered useful in addressing racial disparities in health?

- **a.** Expand knowledge base through data collection and reporting of data by race/ethnicity
- **b.** Improve sources of health financing and care
- **c.** Increase public and provider awareness
- **d.** a and b only
- **e.** All of the above

7. The local health department wishes to eliminate disparities in the receipt of quality care by diabetics and hence narrow the mortality gap between Whites and Blacks in the county. As a director of the minority health office at the health department, which of the following might serve as an effective approach toward narrowing the racial disparities in mortality associated with diabetes in the county?

a. Ensuring that policies direct activities toward diabetes treatment in particular and minority health in general
b. Enhancing research to reduce the disproportionate disease burden in minority groups
c. Developing effective internal and external communication networks
d. b and c only
e. All of the above

8. The consequences of not having private insurance have been persistently evaluated. Health insurance is associated with increased access and utilization of health services. Which of the following should be considered as other consequences of not being insured?

a. Using fewer preventive and screening services
b. Advanced stage at diagnosis of disease
c. Receiving fewer therapeutic services
d. Having poorer health outcomes (higher mortality and disability rates)
e. All of the above

9. Government plays a role in improving the health of the population. Which of the following is (are) considered when enforcing laws and regulations that protect the health of the public?

a. Enforcement of clean air standards
b. Enforcement of sanitary codes
c. Protecting drinking water supplies
d. Animal control
e. All of the above

10. There is disarray in the private health insurance coverage in this nation. Over the years, some solutions have been suggested to address lack of coverage and quality coverage. Which of the following should be considered contributory to addressing the insurance issue?

a. Expanding state programs for low-income people
b. Using taxes to finance a single, national government health plan for all Americans
c. Offering tax credits or other assistance to help businesses provide coverage for employees
d. All of the above
e. None of the above

11. Policy development serves as a core function of public health. The implementation of public health services requires policy development and planning or management. As a public health professional assigned to work with the community to reduce tobacco use, which of the following aspects should be incorporated into your policy development and planning for this project?

a. Systematic community-wide planning for tobacco health improvement
b. Developing and tracking measurable objectives
c. Developing policy and legislation related to the practice of public health in the area of tobacco cessation
d. Implementing joint evaluation with the medical care system in terms of tobacco-related diseases
e. All of the above

12. Public health is charged with disease control and health promotion. This substance reflects the commitment of public health and includes all of the following *except*:

a. Prevention of epidemics and spread of diseases
b. Protection against environmental hazards
c. Assuring the quality and accessibility of health services
d. Responding to disasters and assisting communities in recovery
e. None of the above

13. Public health is charged with monitoring the health status of the population. As a public health professional, what are the activities within this responsibility of public health?

a. Ongoing community health status assessment
b. Identification of threats to health
c. Determination of health service needs
d. a and c only
e. All of the above

14. The framework for examining public health system performance involves capacity, process, and outcomes. The capacity level refers to the input, which involves the interaction with workforce, information, organization and relationships, and facilities and funding. If the process results in the outcome, which of these should be considered as the outcome of public health capacity and process?

a. Improved organizational performance
b. Improved program performance
c. Both of the above
d. Neither of the above

15. The Tuskegee Syphilis Study, conducted from 1932 until 1972, involved 600 subjects (399 cases and 201 controls) and resulted in 28 syphilis-specific deaths, 100 deaths from syphilis-related complications, infection of 40 spouses, and 19 children born with congenital syphilis. This study is an indication of human subject violation in research. Which specific elements in human research conduct were violated by this experiment?

a. Informed consent
b. Right to receive treatment
c. Knowledge of the research
d. Risk inherent in the research
e. All of the above

16. Which of the following international regulations impose(s) ethical duties on researchers who conduct nontherapeutic experiments on human subjects?

a. Helsinki Declaration
b. Nuremberg Code
c. Belmont Code
d. b and c only
e. All of the above

17. The Health Insurance Portability and Accountability Act of 1996 (HIPAA) establishes a federal floor of safeguards to protect the confidentiality of health information. Which of the following statements apply(ies) to this confidentiality act?

a. Regulates uses and disclosures of individually identifiable health information
b. Provides patient rights with respect to their health information
c. Establishes requirements to ensure privacy of patient
d. All of the above
e. None of the above

18. The inclusion of human subjects in research requires approval from the Institutional Review Board (IRB). This approval requires, among other things, an informed consent from all participants. Which of the following is (are) considered substantial in an informed consent?

a. Disclosure of the purpose of the research
b. The benefit of the research in advancing knowledge
c. The risk or harm inherent in the research
d. A statement that participation/consent is voluntary
e. All of the above

19. Policy development is an essential process in fulfilling the requirements of the essential public health services. The formulation of policy often requires communities' mobilization. Which of the following should be considered as essential stages in policy development?

- a. Problem identification
- b. Priority setting
- c. Policy formulation and design
- d. All of the above
- e. None of the above

20. The Institute of Medicine integrated the core functions of public health in its identification of the essential public health services. These services are cyclical and continuous processes managed at the systems level and are enhanced through research. Which of these services are directly linked with policy development?

- a. Mobilizing community partnerships to identify and solve health problems
- b. Enforcing laws and regulations that protect and ensure safety
- c. Health services monitoring and identification of community health needs
- d. Diagnoses and investigation of health problems and health hazards in the community
- e. a and b only

ANNOTATED ANSWERS

1. The correct answer is **E** (health policy and disease prevention).

2. The correct answer is **C** (health policy and the Congress).

3. The correct answer is **E** (health insurance dynamics).

4. The correct answer is **D** (health insurance eligibility).

5. The correct answer is **B** (private health insurance coverage).

6. The correct answer is **E** (racial health disparities elimination).

7. The correct answer is **E** (health disparities narrowing).

8. The correct answer is **E** (health insurance coverage).

9. The correct answer is **E** (enforcing laws and regulations regarding the health of the public).

10. The correct answer is **D** (strategies to improve insurance coverage). Other suggestions include mandating businesses to offer coverage, offering tax credits or other assistance to help purchase private coverage, and expanding Medicare to uninsured under 65 (*Kaiser Family Foundation Health Poll Report*, October 2007).

11. The correct answer is **E** (policy development and planning of public health services). Developing policies and planning involves leadership development at all levels, as well as systematic community-wide planning for tobacco health improvement, developing and tracking measurable objectives, developing policy and legislation related to the practice of public

health in the area of tobacco cessation, and implementing joint evaluation with the medical care system in terms of tobacco-related diseases.

12. The correct answer is **E** (public health services). The commitment of public health also includes injury prevention and the promotion and encouragement of healthy behaviors (Institute of Medicine, *The Future of Public Health*, 1988).

13. The correct answer is **E** (public health responsibility of monitoring health status). Essential public health services include the monitoring of the health status of the population. These activities include (a) attention to special high-risk populations, (b) identification of community assets and resources, (c) interpretation and communication, and (d) management of multi-sectoral information systems. Other aspects of this essential function are (a) ongoing community health status assessment, (b) identification of threats to health, and (c) determination of health service needs.

14. The correct answer is **C** (framework for examining public health system performance).

15. The correct answer is **E** (ethical consideration in research involving human subjects).

16. The correct answer is **B** (human subject in research—international regulation).

17. The correct answer is **D** (HIPAA regulation—Privacy of Individually Identifiable Health Information [PIIHI]).

18. The correct answer is **E** (elements of informed consent). An appropriate informed consent form is required to state the benefits of the research, the qualifications, the affiliations, and the contact information of the principal investigator as well as the IRB that approved the research and the relevant information on the approval. In addition, all informed consent forms must state the risk or harm inherent in the research if applicable, compensation or incentive to be received by participants if applicable, as well as the statement declaring that participation is voluntary; the form must be signed and dated.

19. The correct answer is **D** (policy development stages). Other stages in policy development include (a) passage of policy instruments, (b) implementation, and (c) evaluation.

20. The correct answer is **E** (link between the essential public health services and core functions of public health). The essential public health functions are (a) health services monitoring and identification of community health needs; (b) diagnoses and investigation of health problems and health hazards in the community; (c) informing, educating and empowering people about health issues; (d) mobilizing community partnerships to identify and solve health problems; (e) enforcing laws and regulations that protect and ensure safety; (f) linking people with needed personal health services and ensuring the provision of health care when otherwise unavailable; (g) ensuring a competent public health and personal healthcare workforce; (i) evaluating effectiveness, accessibility, and quality of personal and population-based health services; and (j) researching new insights and innovative solutions to health problems.

Chapter 7

Practice Test

Larry Holmes, Jr.

INSTRUCTIONS AND HINTS

There are 200 questions in this practice test, *all* of which must be attempted. The time allowed is *4.00 hours*, implying that you must spend an average of 72.0 seconds (1.20 minutes) per question. Scientific calculators are allowed and are highly encouraged for this test. There is a higher probability of correctly answering multiple-choice test questions if you apply the following test-taking skills:

1. Attempt the questions that you are most confident of and later return to the ones that present some challenges or are perceived to be more difficult; utilizing the information gained from the less difficult ones can help provide the right answers to the difficult ones.
2. Read the question once, conceive the response and select the right answer. If your conceived response is not among the choices, select the most appropriate after re-reading the question.
3. Attempt the questions that appear to be lengthy last.

Please note that there are obvious incorrect choices. Narrowing your choices by eliminating these obvious incorrect answers increases your chances of obtaining the right answer, thus increasing your yield.

TEST QUESTIONS (MULTIPLE CHOICE)

Directions: Each of the following questions contains multiple suggested responses. Select the *one best* response to each question. Except otherwise specified, most illustrations used in these questions are hypothetical, and have no bearings to any organizations, agencies, institutions, and communities past or present.

1. The substance of public health, its core functions, and its essential services must integrate in the framework of public health performance. Assessment is one of the core functions of public health as declared by the Institute of Medicine. Which of the following activities will be considered in meeting the essential public health services of this core function?

a. Assessment of community health needs
b. Investigation of health hazards and effects
c. Analysis of disease risk factors
d. a and c only
e. All of the above

2. The Institute of Medicine, in *The Future of Public Health* landmark release on the mission and vision of public health, stated categorically that "assurance" is one of the core functions of public health. As a public health professional assigned to a local health department to direct a newly created unit for public health service assurance, which of the following should you expect to be included among your areas of responsibility?

a. Management of resources
b. Implementation of programs
c. Planning and developing policies
d. a and b only
e. All of the above

3. The lessons from the state of California's Tobacco Taxation Program are indicative of the essential role of policy in disease prevention and health promotion. In 1988, Californian Proposition 99 placed a 25¢ tax on cigarette packaging ($90 million per year to change social norms/behavior). Ten years later (1999), there had been a 27% reduction in smoking and a 19% decrease in lung cancer death rates in the state. Therefore, governmental policies such as taxing tobacco to reduce tobacco smoking among youths who are most sensitive to price increases are essential for the improvement of population health. Policy development as a core function of public health embraces all of the following activities *except*:

a. Advocating for community needs and issues
b. Prioritizing health needs
c. Planning and developing policies
d. Evaluating programs
e. None of the above

4. Public health achievement in the 21st century includes motor vehicle safety. During 1925 there were 18 deaths per million vehicle miles traveled (VMT) and in 1997 there were 1.7 deaths per million VMT. The decrease in motor vehicle deaths can be attributed primarily to the public health focus on:

a. Improvements in vehicle safety features
b. Public education on the importance of safety belts
c. Enforcement of traffic laws
d. Improved streets and highways
e. All of the above

5. In 1900, more than 30% of all deaths occurred among children younger than 5 years old, primarily from infectious diseases. Today, that thought is staggering. Public health initiatives such as immunizations, improved sanitation, clean water, and improved food safety have virtually eliminated myriad infectious diseases, including typhoid and cholera—two major causes of illness and death early in the 20th century. Which of the following conditions resulted in safe and healthier food?

a. Refrigeration
b. Pasteurization
c. Healthier animal care, feeding, and processing
d. Improved food supply safety
e. All of the above

6. Compared with the 1900s, average life span has increased in the United States as the direct result of public health initiatives such as vaccinations, sanitation, chlorination, motor vehicle and workplace safety, and improving people's awareness of the importance of healthy lifestyle choices. Which of the following are considered the broad health issues of public health today?

a. Preventing and controlling disease
b. Keeping our environment clean, healthy, and safe
c. Promoting good health practices
d. All of the above
e. None of the above

7. Clinicians may examine men who are diabetic more often or more thoroughly than men who are not. If this observation is accurate, and if an association is observed between erectile dysfunction (ED) and diabetes mellitus in men, the association may be due to which of the following biases?

a. Misclassification bias
b. Recall bias
c. Surveillance bias
d. Interviewer bias
e. None of the above

Questions 8 and 9. A cohort study was conducted to assess the association between incidence of diabetes mellitus type II and exercise, where obesity is assumed to be a confounding factor. Using the accompanying table, answer the following questions.

Exercise Level	DM (Type II)	Person-years	Incidence/ 100,000
All subjects (n = 8,000 person-years)			
Low	105	4,000	
High	25	4,000	6.25
Relative risk			
BMI (> 24.99 kg/m²) (n = 4,000 person-years)			
Low	90	3,000	30.0
High	10	1,000	
Relative risk			
BMI (< 24.99kg/m²) (n = 4,000 person-years)			
Low	15	1,000	
High	15	3,000	5.0
Relative risk			

8. What is the relative risk in low exercise compared with high exercise in all subjects in the study?

a. 3.0
b. 2.3
c. 4.2
d. 2.4
e. Cannot be estimated from the information provided

9. If the relative risk in all subjects differs from the relative risk in the subjects stratified by BMI, which of the following statements may explain this observation?

a. BMI itself is a factor in type II DM
b. BMI is related to exercise
c. BMI is a confounder
d. All of the above
e. None of the above

10. The incidence rate of chronic obstructive pulmonary disease (COPD) in those who smoke is 400 per 10,000 person-years; in those who are exposed to air pollution, it is 200; and in those with neither exposure, it is 40. Estimate the incidence rate in those with both exposures, assuming an additive model.

a. 560 per 10,000 person-years
b. 640 per 10,000 person-years
c. 600 per 10,000 person-years
d. 240 per 10,000 person-years
e. 440 per 10,000 person-years

11. Assuming that smoke and air pollution exert independent effects on COPD in question 10, rendering this joint effect multiplicative, calculate the joint effects of these two variables in the multiplicative model.

a. 1,000 per 10,000
b. 50 per 10,000
c. 2,000 per 10,000
d. 32,000 per 10,000
e. 16,000 per 10,000

12. In a case-control study relating smoking to cancer of the cervix in women, the investigators found the crude odds ratio to be 6.6 and the Mantel–Haenszel odds ratio, adjusted for age, to be 6.3. In addition, their stratified analysis by age indicated the following odds ratio (OR) by the three age groups for smokers, relative to nonsmokers: (a) age 20–29 years, OR = 27.9; (b) age 30–39 years, OR = 5.9; and (c) age 40+, OR = 2.8. Based on these results, age is considered to be a (an):

a. Positive confounder
b. Negative confounder
c. Nuisance covariate
d. Effect measure modifier
e. Confounder

13. Methods for controlling for confounding at the analysis phase of a study include all of the following, *except*:

a. Standardization
b. Randomization
c. Stratified analysis
d. Matched analysis
e. Multivariable analysis

14. All of the following are advantages of prospective cohort study, *except*:

a. Recall bias is minimized compared to case-control designs
b. It is relatively inexpensive compared to case-control design
c. Precise measurement of exposure is possible
d. Incidence rate can be estimated
e. A number of disease outcomes can be studied simultaneously

15. The accompanying table presents the age group, number of person-years, and the mortality rate in standard population.

Age Group	Number of Person-years	Mortality Rate in Standard Population per 100,000	Expected Number of Deaths
25–34	7,557	0.8	
35–44	4,023	4.8	
45–54	2,961	47.9	
55–64	2,043	265.8	

If the total observed mortality from lung cancer is 12, what is the standardized mortality ratio?

- a. 7.10
- b. 12.0
- c. 0.59
- d. 1.69
- e. Cannot be estimated from the information on the table

16. Regarding a case-control design, all of the following are accurate, *except*:

- a. Recall bias is a potential problem
- b. It is possible to have multiple comparison groups
- c. Disease rates are compared for subjects with the factor of interest and for those without the factor of interest
- d. The proportion of cases with exposure is compared with the proportion of controls with the exposure
- e. The odds ratio is the measure of the association

17. Which of the following is *correct* regarding ecologic fallacy?

- **a.** Occurs when assessing exposure in large groups rather than small groups
- **b.** Occurs when assessing outcomes in large groups rather than in small groups
- **c.** Occurs due to the investigator's inability to assess temporal sequence in causal inference
- **d.** Occurs when an investigator attributes the characteristics of a group to every individual in the group
- **e.** None of the above

18. An observational study (case-control) was conducted to determine the association between male hormones (testosterone, dihydrotestosterone, sex hormone-bidding globulin, and androstenidione) and prostate cancer among 1,850 U.S. residents aged 45 years and older. The investigators observed dihydrotestosterone as a risk for prostate cancer with an odds ratio of 2.6. What are the possible explanations for this finding?

- **a.** Causal association
- **b.** Chance association
- **c.** Spurious association
- **d.** a and c only
- **e.** All of the above

19. The mortality rate in population A differs from the mortality rate in population B based on the crude comparison. Epidemiologists often utilize age-adjusted rates. This rate is used to:

- **a.** Assess the coefficient of determination of mortalities in the populations
- **b.** Correct the death rates for errors in the statement of age
- **c.** Determine the actual number of deaths that occur in specific age groups
- **d.** Remove the effects of differences in the age distributions of populations in comparing death rates
- **e.** Compare the relative risk of dying in the two populations

20. The prevalence of a disease is an indication of the status of a disease in the population and does not provide information on the cause of the disease. The incidence of the disease reflects the new cases of the disease in a population. There is relationship between the prevalence and the incidence of the disease as well as the duration. If the incidence rate of gout is 5 times greater in women than in men, but the prevalence proportion indicates no sex difference, which of the following statements is *most* accurate?

a. The case fatality rate for gout is greater for women
b. The crude all-cause mortality rate is greater for women
c. The case fatality rate for gout is lower for women
d. The duration of gout is shorter in men
e. The predisposing factors for gout are more common in women

21. In a case-control study of osteoporosis, investigators examined 100 women as case and an equal number of women as control and found low-calcium intake in 40 of the cases and 20 of the controls. What is the odds ratio in the association between low-calcium intake and developing osteoporosis in this population?

a. 1.53
b. 15.3
c. 2.66
d. 26.6
e. Cannot be estimated from the information provided

22. In a trial of an antiretroviral drug for AIDS treatment, the investigators reported 4 deaths among 55 patients treated with this agent, compared with 14 deaths among 52 controls on placebo. Calculate the attributable benefit of this agent in reducing mortality associated with AIDS in this study population.

a. 19.6%
b. 1.96%
c. 7.3%
d. 26.9%
e. 1.93%

23. Clinical trial is considered a gold standard in terms of epidemiologic designs. The purpose of random assignment in clinical trial is to:

a. Minimize selection bias in the allocation of treatment
b. Enhance double blinding
c. Facilitate the measurement of the exposure variables
d. Facilitate the measurement of the outcome variable
e. Control for confounding (comparable baseline characteristics)

24. Double-blind design is often used in clinical trials. The purpose of double masking or blinding in these studies is to:

a. Minimize sampling error
b. Minimize interviewer bias
c. Minimize confounding due to observation
d. Ensure comparability of treated (treatment) and untreated (control) subjects
e. Reduce the effects of surveillance bias

25. A case-control design selects subjects based on disease, whereas cohort design selects subjects on the basis of exposure. Which of the following is a case-control study?

a. A study of cancer in men who have quit smoking
b. A study of the incidence of osteoporosis in women with low-calcium injection
c. Obtaining histories and other information from a group of known cases and a comparison group to determine the relative frequency of exposure under study
d. Study of proportionate mortality using cumulative cases
e. Analysis of previous research in order to establish summary point estimate

26. Epidemiologic causal inference relies on some set of criteria, especially those of Bradford Hill and Richard Doll. Which of the following is *inaccurate* when making causal inference using Hill's criteria?

a. Positive predictive value
b. Strength of association
c. Dose-response relationship
d. Temporality
e. Specificity

27. Bias is a systematic error arising from inaccurate measurement. Compared with prospective cohort study, which of the following biases is *most* commonly associated with case-control design?

a. Interviewer bias
b. Surveillance bias
c. Recall bias
d. Lead time bias
e. Nonresponse bias

28. Which of the following statements is (are) concerning confounding?

a. Distortion of an exposure-outcome association is due to the association of another factor with both outcome and exposure
b. To be a confounding, a factor has to be independently associated with both exposure and the outcome under consideration
c. Both of the above
d. Neither of the above

29. Regarding recall bias:

- **a.** Occurs when the level of accuracy differs between the compared groups
- **b.** Occurs in case-control studies when cases remember or report information differently from control
- **c.** Occurs in prospective cohort study when individuals who are exposed remember/report subsequent illnesses differently than those who are unexposed
- **d.** a and c only
- **e.** All of the above

30. Sources of epidemiologic data include all the following, *except*:

- **a.** Vital statistics
- **b.** National Health and Nutrition Examination Survey
- **c.** National Health Interview Survey
- **d.** Behavioral Risk Factors Surveillance Systems
- **e.** None of the above

31. Which of the following statements is *correct* concerning cross-sectional study?

- **a.** Examines the rate of disease in relation to population-level factor
- **b.** The unit of analysis is population rather than individual
- **c.** Defines subjects according to exposure level and follows them for disease occurrence
- **d.** Defines cases of disease and controls and compares the exposure histories
- **e.** Cannot infer the temporal sequence between the exposure and disease

32. In a country with a population of 3 million people, 30,000 deaths occurred during the year ending December 31, 2005. These included 15,000 deaths from malaria in 50,000 people who were sick with malaria. What was the case-fatality rate from malaria in 2005?

a. 0.3%
b. 30%
c. 33.3%
d. 1.0%

33. A graduate student is expected to interpret the study on the association between breast cancer and high-fat diet. In the process of preparing his/her defense for the interpretation, s/he wishes to reflect on chance variation (random error), observation bias (systematic error), and confounding (the mixing effect of an external factor on the association between high-fat diet and breast cancer). Which of the following should s/he consider *first* in the interpretation of the study?

a. Confounding
b. Random error
c. Observation (measurement) bias
d. a and c simultaneously
e. None of the above

34. Which of the following measures expresses the degree to which risk for a specific outcome is due to a specific exposure?

a. Absolute risk
b. Absolute risk increase
c. Absolute risk reduction
d. Attributable risk percent
e. Attributable risk

35. Publication bias is one of the issues confronting the use of the interpretation from meta-analysis for decision-making regarding interventions. Which of the following is accurate regarding publication bias in the conduct of meta-analysis?

a. Exists if the results of a study influence whether it is published or presented, or whether it is easily retrieved
b. The most likely effect of publication bias is that small studies that show strong, significant, or unusual results are more likely to be published than small studies that show null results or results in the expected direction
c. Both of the above
d. Neither of the above

36. A fixed-effect meta-analysis was conducted to examine the overall survival benefit of long-term versus short-term androgen deprivation therapy (ADT). The authors reported a hazard ratio (HR) of 0.52, 95% CI = 0.39–0.68, and chi square (χ^2) for homogeneity test of 4.5, with 4 degrees of freedom, $p = 0.4$. Which of the following interpretations could be made from these data?

a. Compared with short-term ADT, long-term ADT significantly increased overall survival by 48%
b. Compared with short-term ADT, long-term ADT significantly increased overall survival by 52%
c. Compared with short-term ADT, long-term ADT nonsignificantly increased overall survival by 48%
d. Compared with short -term ADT, long-term ADT nonsignificantly increased overall survival by 52%
e. None of the above

37. Public health needs to help communities increase access to safe, nutritious food grown in a sustainable way so that people can make healthy food choices. Such public health efforts can contribute to the prevention and control of which of the following ailments or conditions?

a. Obesity
b. Diabetes
c. Cancer
d. Heart disease
e. All of the above

38. Health policy is a multidimensional process. Which of the following statements is (are) *correct* regarding the role of the Congress in U.S. health policy?

a. Congress plays an integral role in the development, financing, and oversight of public and private sector health policies
b. Congressional health policy agenda are driven by a range of forces, including the presidential budget, political agenda, lobbying, and advocacy
c. Both of the above
d. Neither of the above

39. More than 60% of nonelderly Americans get private health insurance at work as a benefit from their own job or as the spouse or dependent of a working family member. Data have consistently shown that having private insurances increases the risk for late diagnosis from melanoma, prostate, and breast cancer. Which of the following conditions may result in a change in insurance coverage?

a. Loss of job
b. Change in family status
c. Birthday
d. Change in health status
e. All of the above

40. Private insurance through employer differs from individual insurance. Which of the following statements is (are) indicative of the basic distinction?

a. Eligibility is not based on health status in individual insurance
b. Eligibility is based on age and health status in employer-sponsored insurance
c. Both of the above
d. Neither of the above

41. Private health insurance coverage is not a right but a service for those who can afford it. All of the following are true regarding coverage, *except*:

a. Private insurance is a mainstay of health coverage for most Americans, but access, affordability, and adequacy of coverage are not guaranteed
b. Despite limited access to coverage, disease prognosis is not related by any known study or research to insurance coverage
c. The difficulty of getting/keeping private coverage increases with health problems, especially during coverage transitions
d. Regulation to limit risk selection involves trade-offs: access versus adequacy versus affordability
e. Additional public policy responses are needed to subsidize and expand coverage

42. The Healthy People 2010 objective indicates the need to eliminate health disparities. Which of the following strategies should be considered useful in addressing racial disparities in health?

a. Expand the knowledge base through data collection and reporting of data by race/ethnicity
b. Improve sources of health financing and care
c. Increase public and provider awareness
d. a and b only
e. All of the above

43. The local health department wishes to eliminate disparities in the receipt of quality care by diabetics and hence narrow the mortality gap between Whites and Blacks in the county. As a director of the minority health office at the health department, which of the following might serve as an effective approach toward narrowing the racial disparities in mortality associated with diabetes in the county?

a. Ensuring that policies direct activities toward diabetes treatment in particular and minority health in general
b. Enhancing research to reduce the disproportionate disease burden in minority groups
c. Developing effective internal and external communication networks
d. b and c only
e. All of the above

44. The consequences of not having private insurance have been persistently evaluated. Health insurance is associated with increased access and utilization of health services. Which of the following should be considered as other consequences of not being insured?

a. Using fewer preventive and screening services
b. Advanced stage at diagnosis of disease
c. Receiving fewer therapeutic services
d. Having poorer health outcomes (higher mortality and disability rates)
e. All of the above

45. Government plays a role in improving the health of the population. Which of the following is (are) considered under enforcing laws and regulations that protect the health of the public?

a. Enforcement of clean air standards
b. Enforcement of sanitary codes
c. Protecting drinking water supplies
d. Animal control
e. All of the above

46. There is disarray in private health insurance coverage in this nation. Over the years, some solutions have been suggested to address lack of coverage and quality coverage. Which of the following are considered contributory to addressing the insurance issue?

- **a.** Expanding state programs for low-income people
- **b.** Using taxes to finance a single, national government health plan for all Americans
- **c.** Offering tax credits or other assistance to help businesses provide coverage for employees
- **d.** All of the above
- **e.** None of the above

47. The bio-psychosocial model of health, which focuses on the multifactorial causes of disease, could be applied to which of the following conditions as an attempt to understand their etio-pathogenesis?

- **a.** Cardiovascular disorders
- **b.** Cancer
- **c.** Diabetes
- **d.** a and c only
- **e.** All of the above

48. An investigator is interested in a behavioral intervention that will increase self-efficacy in the participants. In which of the following conditions will self-efficacy be an effective intervention model in reducing the behavioral risk and maintain healthful behaviors?

- **a.** Smoking
- **b.** Sexual behavior
- **c.** Drug abuse
- **d.** b and c only
- **e.** All of the above

49. The potential for biological, chemical, and nuclear agents to be used in a terrorist attack, has received wide publicity in the United States since September 11, 2001. However, the role of public health through behavioral sciences in attempting to understand the present terrorists threats and concerns with the immediate and long-term behavioral consequences of terrorism remains unclear. As a public health professional, what will you consider to be the main purpose(s) of terrorism?

- a. Instill fear in the population
- b. Change the behavior of governments
- c. Compress mortality
- d. a and b only
- e. All of the above

50. A survey study conducted to examine the emerging risk factors in diabetes mellitus in New-town, No-State, revealed excessive inactivity as one of the exposure (independent/predictor) variables. As a public health professional, you are expected to implement an intervention to increase physical activities in this population. The strategies for this behavior change will include:

- a. Individual
- b. Group
- c. Community
- d. Technology-based
- e. All of the above

51. Social and economic factors are major determinants of health. Which of the following statements is (are) correct regarding the observed role of this factor in disease progression and prognosis?

- a. The quality of the social environment is worse where financial deprivation is greatest, such as the inner cities
- b. The ill effects due to absolute poverty, meaning societies in which there is a wide gap between the rich and the poor, suffer additional social problems, for instance, through high rates of violence, crime, and truancy

c. People with good social networks live longer, are at reduced risk of coronary heart disease, are less likely to report being depressed or to suffer a recurrence of cancer, and are less susceptible to infectious illness than those with poor networks
d. a and b only
e. All of the above

52. The life expectancy gained in the U.S. population has been attributed to behavior changes at the population level toward tobacco cessation practices. This has resulted in dramatic decreases in heart diseases and stroke. Tobacco remains the leading predisposing factor to death in the United States, accounting for 18.1% of the total predisposing factors and conditions associated with death. Which of the following health conditions is (are) associated with smoking?

a. Lung, mouth, and throat cancers
b. Chronic obstructive pulmonary disease
c. Renal cancer
d. a and c only
e. All of the above

53. The ecologic model of health behavior proposes the role of social environment in the implementation of an effective health promotion and disease prevention program. As a public health department, the City Health Department wishes to reduce the obesity epidemic among inner-city Hispanic males by using the ecologic model. Which of the following stages will be essential in your implementation?

a. Intrapersonal factors
b. Interpersonal factors
c. Institutional factors
d. Community factors
e. Public policy
f. a, c, and e only
g. All of the above

54. During the past three decades, a great deal of research has been focused on how to increase people's self-efficacy, thereby helping motivate them to practice healthy behaviors. As a proponent of this model of behavior change, which of the following examples would you consider adequate in increasing self-efficacy?

- **a.** Previous successful performance
- **b.** Role-modeling
- **c.** Small-group exercise
- **d.** Skills practice
- **e.** All of the above
- **f.** None of the above

55. Studies on psychological and social factors that influence health have consistently implicated stress and social support in the outcome of disease and mortality. Which of the following statements support the role played by stress in disease prognosis and mortality?

- **a.** Widows and widowers tend to have an unusually high risk of dying soon after the death of their spouse
- **b.** Mortality rates of survivors are 40% to 50% higher during the 6 months after the death of a spouse relative to the mortality of married people of the same age
- **c.** People who lose their jobs are 50% to 70% more likely to present with angina symptoms compared to their employed counterparts of the same age and similar sociodemographics
- **d.** a and c only
- **e.** All of the above

56. Race and ethnicity are consistently shown to influence disease prevalence and mortality in the United States, and ethnic minorities, particularly Blacks, tend to be disproportionately affected and bear the burden of most diseases in the nation. Because race/ethnicity is a complex phenomenon, which of the following demographic variations may explain the observed burden of morbidity and mortality of Blacks relative to Whites?

- **a.** Income
- **b.** Education
- **c.** Occupation
- **d.** a and c only
- **e.** All of the above

57. Social support network has been found to be strongly associated with an individual's health status and risk of dying. This association is observed to be true for both genders, regardless of socioeconomic status. Because absence of social support or contact has been associated with an increase in coronary heart disease, pregnancy complications, and prematurity and infant mortality, which of the following statements provide a possible explanation for the observed associations?

- **a.** Social contact is effective in stress buffering
- **b.** Relaxation may be achieved through social contacts and social support networks
- **c.** Social contact increases adrenal gland secretion, releasing excessive dopamine and norepinephrine, thus reducing stress
- **d.** Social contact my potentiate the immune responsiveness, thus serving as a protective mechanism for tissue inflammation and repair
- **e.** a, b, and d only

58. The health belief model of behavior change assumes that humans act in rational ways and are more likely to change behavior when confronted with a threat. If you are assigned to the Breast Cancer Prevention Program (BCPP) and wish to use this model in promoting breast self-examination among Asian-American women, which of the following factors will you consider in your implementation of this model?

a. The extent to which Asian-American women feel vulnerable to breast cancer
b. The perceived severity of breast cancer
c. The perceived effectiveness of taking action to prevent or minimize breast cancer as compared to barriers to and costs of taking such an action
d. All of the above
e. None of the above

59. Interventions to address risky behaviors such as smoking cessation, poor dietary patterns, and physical inactivity have been shown to be efficacious. These studies have utilized standard methodology to determine the efficacy of intervention studies. As a public health professional, if you wish to replicate or translate these proven interventions to your community in determining their effectiveness, which of the following aspects of community-based intervention will you consider?

a. Population that might benefit most from the intervention
b. Which location or agent would work best in the implementation
c. How many people would choose to use a program that has not been fully evaluated
d. All of the above
e. None of the above

60. The basis of behavioral intervention is the consistent indication of behavior change. Which of the following statements is inaccurate concerning behavior change?

a. Behavioral interventions can successfully teach new behavior
b. Behavioral interventions are solely designed to potentiate risky behaviors
c. Behavioral interventions can successfully attenuate risky behaviors
d. Maintaining behavior over time is a greater challenge
e. Short-term changes in behavior are encouraging, but improved health outcomes will often require prolonged interventions and lengthy follow-up

61. Research efforts to elucidate the mechanisms by which social and psychological factors influence health are essential to health promotions and disease prevention. Which of the following is (are) *correct* regarding behavioral intervention?

a. Intervention studies are needed to evaluate the efficacy and effectiveness of modifying health risk behaviors
b. Intervention studies should span the breath of all phases of clinical trials, from feasibility studies to randomized double-blinded studies
c. Intervention should include all levels of participants, from individual to family, community, and society
d. All of the above
e. None of the above

62. All of the following are correct concerning intervention strategy, *except*:

a. Concurrent intervention at multiple levels should not be encouraged as this will not lead to the promotion of healthy behaviors
b. Behavioral and psychosocial interventions should be long term for optimal outcome
c. Individual behavior, family interactions, community and workplace relationships, resources, and public policy all contribute to health and influence behavior change
d. Interventions at multiple levels (individual, family, community, society) are more likely to sustain behavioral change
e. Interventions should address psychosocial factors associated with health status such as access to healthy food and safe places to exercise, as well as individual behavior

63. Changing unhealthy behavior is not simply a matter of "willpower." Individual behavior has biological underpinnings and consequences and is influenced by the social and psychological contexts in which it occurs. Which of the following changes is (are) necessary for improvement and maintenance of population health?

a. Social factors
b. Policies
c. Norms
d. All of the above
e. a and c only

64. Obesity is next to tobacco in terms of the population's burden of disease. This condition is dramatically increasing and has become epidemic in the United States. All of the following health risk behaviors or conditions are linked to this epidemic, *except*:

a. Excessive caloric intake
b. Inadequate physical activity
c. Diabetes
d. Birth defects
e. Osteoporosis

65. Interventions at individual and group levels have been conducted to reduce HIV risk behaviors among the most vulnerable and populations at highest risk in the United States. In spite of these interventions, African-American women remain the fastest growing segment of incident AIDS cases. Obviously, new research is needed to provide intervention at individual, family, community, and society levels. As an HIV/AIDS interventionist, which of the following factors will you consider as HIV/AIDS-related behavior to incorporate into your model in reducing HIV risky behaviors?

a. Knowledge
b. Subjective norms
c. Perceived risk
d. Self-efficacy
e. All of the above

66. Smoking behavior tends to follow some socio-demographic patterns. Which of the following findings or statements support such observed pattern?

a. The prevalence of smoking among blue-collar workers is higher compared with the while-collar workers
b. Compared with Whites or Blacks, American Indians and Alaskan Natives smoke at much higher rates
c. The prevalence rate of smoking is higher among men with less than high school education compared with male and female college students of the same age
d. All of the above
e. None of the above

67. The Behavioral Risk Factor Surveillance System (BRFSS) is a source of data for health risk behaviors in chronic and infectious diseases. The Youth Risk Behavior Survey is another source of data for health risk factors. This dataset characterizes the prevalence of selected health-risk behaviors among adolescents aged 12 to 19 years who do and do not attend school. Which of the following findings serve to support the role of education in health-risk behaviors?

- **a.** In-school adolescents are significantly more likely to have reported "always" using safety belts while riding in a car or truck, relative to out-of-school adolescents
- **b.** In-school adolescent are less likely to report driving under the influence of alcohol
- **c.** Out-of-school adolescents are significantly less likely to use marijuana or cocaine
- **d.** All of the above
- **e.** None of the above

68. Public health researchers should consider the particular study design being used in their survey and the type of research questions that can be addressed with the design. Some of the commonly used designs in studying health-risk behaviors include cross-sectional or group comparison, longitudinal designs, and experimental designs. Essential to longitudinal design is predictive criteria, implying the prediction of changes over time. Which of the following statements is (are) *true* regarding this design (longitudinal)?

- **a.** Variations in the health indicator may be affected by other external factors in the environment
- **b.** Changes in the questions in the successive waves of study could introduce errors in detecting true changes in these indicators over time
- **c.** Improvement in diagnostic and treatment modalities or techniques for a selected illness can lead to a higher survival, thus a higher prevalence of the disease over time
- **d.** a and b only
- **e.** All of the above

69. Multiple regression procedures may be used when two or more interval-level measures serve as predictors of some normally distributed interval-level dependent variable. In this model, the regression coefficient for any particular independent or explanatory variable (X_1) represents the change in the response or dependent variable (Y) associated with a one-unit change in X_1, while controlling for or maintaining other predictors (X_2, X_3, etc.) at constant. If required to use this predictive model in the analysis of a study data, which of the following assumptions is (are) necessary for a valid result?

- **a.** The dependent variable should be normally distributed around the prediction line
- **b.** Interval or ratio scaled are appropriate
- **c.** Both of the above
- **d.** Neither of the above

70. A study was conducted to examine the differences in average cholesterol level of Black and Asian children (X_1), while controlling for poverty status (X_2). If the analytic method used here is the two-way analysis of variance, which of the following statements is (are) *correct* regarding this technique?

- **a.** An *F*-test statistic can be used to summarize the difference in the variances between and within Black and Asian children on the dependent variable (Y)
- **b.** The greater the variance between Black and Asian children, compared with the variance within Black children and the variance within Asian children, the more likely it is that the differences in cholesterol level between Black and Asian children are statistically significant
- **c.** Both of the above
- **d.** Neither of the above

71. The chi square statistic is often used in behavioral data to test for relationships between variables. This procedure is based on the null hypothesis of no association or independence. Which of the following statements is (are) correct regarding this analytic technique?

a. It is a nonparametric procedure involving nominal data
b. It examines the difference between the distribution that is observed and the distribution that would be expected, assuming the variables are not related
c. The less the variance between the observed and expected, the less support there is for the null hypothesis that there is no relationship between the variable in the particular sample
d. a and c only
e. All of the above

72. Obesity intervention often utilized community trials to increase physical activity. These trials are usually part of a "Healthy Heart" program and incorporate social and environmental measures, including public service announcements about physical activity and total well-being. This approach in terms of health behavior model is best described as the:

a. Transtheoretical Model
b. Health Belief Model
c. Social Support Model
d. Ecologic Model
e. Information, Motivation, and Skill Building Model

73. Recent investigations on the overall health of the U.S. population indicated improvement over the past decades. However, health disparities among racial and ethnic minorities have persisted. Which of the following statements support these findings?

a. Life expectancy in 2001 was 77.7 years for Whites and 72.2 years for Blacks
b. African-American women in 2006 represent an estimated 70% of total incident AIDS cases among women
c. Infant mortality rate for Blacks in 2001 was 2.3 times higher than that of Whites
d. All of the above
e. None of the above

74. Effective behavior intervention transcends individuals and involves families, groups, and public policy. Which of the following illustrates the influence of policy in behavior change?

a. Raising tobacco taxes
b. Company's reduction of the price of cigarettes
c. Restrictions on advertising and promotion
d. a and c only
e. None of the above

75. Infant mortality has declined in the Unites States over the past decade due to improved socioeconomic status, housing, nutrition, immunization, clean water and pasteurized milk, antibiotics, and prenatal and delivery care. The specific causes differ by race, with the leading cause of infant mortality for Whites being congenital anomalies and for Blacks, prematurity and low birth weight. Which of the following factors may help explain the variation in the race-specific etiology of infant mortality?

a. Lower socioeconomic status of African Americans
b. Out-of-wedlock birth of African Americans
c. Young maternal age and low maternal education of African Americans
d. Maternal alcohol consumption of White Americans
e. All of the above

76. One of the conditions for the efficacy of a behavioral intervention is the duration of intervention and the immunization of loss to follow-up or retention. Which of these intervention models of behavior change *explicitly* claims a high degree of retention of subjects?

a. Health Belief
b. Information Motivation and Skill Building
c. Transtheoretical
d. Theory of Reasoned Action
e. Social Cognitive

77. The therapeutic effect of Isotretinoin (Accutane) in treating acne has been documented. Accutane is a Vitamin A derivative, and large doses of Vitamin A are known to be teratogenic. Which of the following statements support(s) the role of Accutane as a teratogen?

a. Of women using Accutane during pregnancy, 20% have given birth to a defective child
b. Accutane received FDA approval with the stipulation that it is contraindicated during pregnancy
c. Both of the above
d. Neither of the above

78. Transport is the dominant source of air pollution in urban areas, with a large part of the urban population still being exposed to excesses of ambient quality levels for one or more pollutants. Which of the following is (are) a known source of air pollution associated with transport?

a. Particulate matter
b. Nitrogen dioxide
c. Benzene
d. Ozone
e. All of the above

79. Long-term, low-level exposure electromagnetic fields may cause adverse health effects via "chronic" impacts, or otherwise influence people's well-being. Scientific knowledge about the health effects of electromagnetic fields (EMF) is substantial and is based on a large number of epidemiological, animal, and in vitro studies. Many health outcomes have been examined. Which of the following health outcomes have been consistently linked with EMF?

a. Reproductive defects
b. Cardiovascular
c. Neuro-degenerative diseases
d. Childhood leukemia
e. None of the above

80. Toxic substances are often described by their abilities to cause adverse or unwanted health effects. Which of the following statements describes risk?

a. Capacity of a substance to cause an adverse effect in a specific organ or organ system
b. Probability that a hazard will occur under specific exposure conditions
c. Weighing of policy alternatives and selection of the most appropriate regulatory actions
d. A statistically derived probability that an adverse effect will occur at a defined exposure level
e. None of the above

81. In the risk assessment process, the hazard identification step performs which of the following functions?

a. Characterizes the relation between doses and incidences of adverse effects in exposed populations
b. Measures or estimates the intensity, frequency, and duration of human exposures to agents
c. Characterizes the innate adverse toxic effects of agents
d. Is the first step in the risk assessment process
e. None of the above

82. What data are most desirable to identify the primary hazard in the hazard identification step?

a. Animal bioassay data
b. Supporting data from cell and biochemical studies
c. Human epidemiology data
d. All of the above
e. None of the above

83. The structure-activity relationship (SAR) has value in risk assessments in that it:

a. Can often be used to predict possible toxicity
b. Is used to design cell studies of the chemical's metabolism
c. Can identify damage to DNA by actual testing of its chemical activity and biochemical structure
d. Has value in risk assessments in that it can often be used to predict possible toxicity
e. None of the above

84. The EPA classification of a substance as a "probable human carcinogen" requires that the substance meet which of the following criteria?

a. Inadequate evidence of cancer in humans and sufficient evidence of cancer in animals
b. Limited evidence of cancer in animals
c. Sufficient human evidence for a causal association between exposure and cancer
d. Inadequate evidence in humans
e. None of the above

85. The primary toxic effect that determines the type of procedure to be used in conducting a risk assessment is:

a. Lethality in laboratory animals
b. Evidence that the chemical is noncarcinogenic
c. The ability of the chemical to cause eye irritation
d. Evidence that the chemical is carcinogenic
e. None of the above

86. Although pesticides are used specifically to kill pets, many of them have environmental impacts as well as toxic effects on humans. The environmental impact of their use includes resistance development, killing of beneficial species, and environmental contaminants. Which of the following is (are) the result(s) of unintended contamination by pesticides?

a. Direct killing of organisms exposed to chemicals
b. Indirect killing via depletion of food or habitat
c. Groundwater contamination
d. Indirect contamination via food chains
e. All of the above

87. The primary method used to predict movement of substances in environmental media is:

a. Actual measurements of air and water pollutants at various places in the environment
b. Use of exposure models
c. Tagging pollutants with radioactive tracers and measuring the radioactivity at various times and locations within the environmental media
d. Exposure models that are the primary method used to predict movement of substances in environmental media
e. None of the above

88. Exposure assessment is a key phase in the risk assessment process because without an exposure, even the most toxic chemical does not present a threat. Which of the following steps is (are) included in the exposure assessment?

a. Characterization of the exposure setting (e.g., point source)
b. Identification of exposure pathways (e.g., groundwater)
c. Quantification of the exposure (e.g., μg/L water)
d. All of the above
e. None of the above

89. The main factors in the exposure assessment are:

a. Exposed populations (general public or selected groups)
b. Types of substances (pharmaceuticals, occupational chemicals, or environmental pollutants)
c. Duration of exposure (brief, intermittent, or protracted)
d. Pathways and media (ingestion, inhalation, and dermal exposure)
e. All of the above

90. A major aspect of the exposure assessment is to:

a. Determine the amount of exposure that must be reduced in order to comply with the acceptable risk level
b. Identify the exposure pathways
c. Measure the amount of a substance that is metabolized in the body
d. All of the above
e. None of the above

91. When actual measurements of exposures are often not available, exposure models may be used. Which of the following is (are) considered as exposure pathways?

a. Groundwater
b. Air
c. Food

d. Breast milk
e. All of the above

92. The process in which the dose-response assessment and exposure assessments are integrated to predict risk in specific populations is known as:

a. Risk management
b. Hazard identification
c. Risk characterization
d. Risk modification
e. Risk quantification

93. An increased cancer risk of 2.0×10^{-6} means that:

a. It is likely that 2 persons in 1 million will develop the specific type of cancer in their lifetime due to exposure to the chemical
b. The xenobiotic for which the cancer risk assessment was performed is likely to cause cancer in 200 persons on a yearly basis
c. It is probable that 2 million persons will develop cancer if they are continuously exposed to the chemical for life
d. a and c only
e. None of the above

94. Power plants, factories, and vehicles spew out harmful gases and small particles that can penetrate deep into human lungs, causing health problems. In strong sunlight, oxides of nitrogen from vehicle exhaust fumes form ozone at ground level, which can trigger asthma attacks. Which of the following constitute(s) major outdoor pollutants that can have an adverse effect on human health?

a. Particulate matter
b. Ozone
c. Carbon monoxide
d. a and c only
e. All of the above

95. Parental smoking and indoor and outdoor air pollutants have been associated with childhood asthma, and asthma is one of the leading causes of chronic disease among children. Which of the following is (are) indicative of increases in asthma severity among children with the condition?

a. Frequency and intensity of asthma attack
b. Number of emergency room visits during the year
c. Occurrence of asthma attacks that require intubations
d. a and b only
e. All of the above

96. Health consequences of secondhand tobacco smoke have been persistently observed. There is biological plausibility of exposure to secondhand smoke causing adverse neurodevelopment effects in children whose parents smoke. Which of the following statements is (are) adequate concerning health effects of secondhand smoke?

a. Gaseous components of secondhand tobacco smoke may adversely affect lung defenses with an effect on cilia and macrophage functions
b. Secondhand tobacco smoke may increase the severity of acute respiratory illness by irritating and inflaming the lungs
c. Secondhand tobacco smoke may contribute to eustachian tube dysfunction through a decrease in mucocilliary clearance, an increase in adenoidal hyperplasia, and an increase in mucosal swelling
d. a and c only
e. All of the above

97. Particle size is the most important factor in determining where particles are deposited in the lung. Deposition of fine particles in distal airways may cause:

a. Acute respiratory morbidity (pneumonia, asthma)
b. Increased mortality (from all causes)
c. Decreased lung function in children

d. All of the above
e. None of the above

98. Several toxic substances affect air quality. Some express their effect on indoor air quality, whereas others on outdoor air quality. Which of the following is (are) a major source of indoor air pollution?

a. Coal and biomass fuel
b. Suspended particulate matter
c. Carbon monoxide and other toxic gases
d. Secondhand tobacco smoke
e. All of the above

99. Toxic substances associated with indoor air pollutants can cause acute health consequences. Which of the following acute conditions is (are) *expected* to be associated with indoor air pollutants?

a. Irritation of the mucous membranes
b. Increased airway responsiveness to allergens
c. Decreased incidence of acute respiratory illness
d. a and b only
e. All of the above

100. Toxic substances associated with indoor air pollutants can cause chronic health effects. Which of the following chronic conditions is (are) *expected* to be associated with long-term exposure to indoor air pollutants?

a. Decreased lung growth
b. Impairment of pulmonary function
c. Increased susceptibility to chronic obstructive lung diseases, including asthma
d. All of the above
e. None of the above

101. Carbon monoxide (CO) is implicated as a potent and lethal air pollutant. Which of the following is (are) considered as the major source(s) of CO?

a. Gas, kerosene, wood stoves, and coal
b. Fireplaces and furnaces
c. Tobacco smoke
d. Vehicle exhaust in a closed garage
e. All of the above

102. The clinical features of CO poisoning are highly variable, and symptoms vary from mild to very severe. As an environmental health specialist for the county's health department, you are at a scene with individuals exposed to CO. Which of the following manifestations would you expect to observe?

a. Dizziness, fatigue, dyspnea
b. Vomiting
c. Irritability
d. Unconsciousness, coma
e. All of the above

103. CO intoxication or poisoning carries lethal consequences. What are the primary prevention modalities that may help reduce the poisoning and mortality associated with CO?

a. Limiting exposure to known CO sources
b. Proper installation, maintenance, and use of combustion appliances
c. Both of the above
d. Neither of the above

104. Cigarette smoking during pregnancy has been associated with congenital anomalies. Which of the following statements support the role of smoking during pregnancy and children's health?

a. Children whose mothers smoke have more respiratory problems than children whose mothers do not smoke
b. Pneumonia and hospitalization in the first year of life is more frequent in children whose mothers smoke
c. Infant mortality is higher in children born to women who smoked during pregnancy than in children of nonsmokers
d. Infants of mothers who smoke have a higher risk of sudden infant death syndrome (SIDS) than infants of mothers who do not smoke
e. All of the above

105. Molds are biologic pollutants and are associated with many health issues in the U.S. population. Which of the following conditions may be described as mold related?

a. Airway and conjunctival irritation
b. Hypersensitivity reactions such as asthma and rhinitis
c. Infections due to immunologic reactions or effects
d. a and b only
e. All of the above

106. Mycotoxins are elaborated by mold and are associated with human disease and cause acute and chronic effects. Which of the following mold toxins is (are) described as hepatotoxins and is (are) carcinogenic?

a. Tricothecenes
b. Ochratoxins
c. Citrinin
d. Aflatoxins
e. All of the above

107. The Sick Building Syndrome has been associated with loss of productivity at the workplace due to frequency absence from work by employees. As an environmental public health specialist expected to increase work attendance and hence productivity to improve the overall life quality of your community, which of the following should be considered as possible solutions to reduce the incidence of Sick Building Syndrome?

a. Removing the source of pollutant
b. Increasing ventilation
c. Cleaning and changing air filters
d. Education and communication
e. All of the above

108. Radon is a radioactive gas released from soil and rocks and is second only to cigarette smoke as a carcinogenic substance in lung cancer. The radon migration system includes:

a. Gas-permeable layer
b. Plastic sheeting
c. Sealing and caulking
d. Vent pipe
e. Junction box
f. All of the above

109. The effects of exposure are influenced by individual susceptibility, which depends on age, developmental stage, nutrition, and social support. Pollutants in the indoor environment are potentially more hazardous to children than adults because their lungs are still growing and maturing; younger children breathe more air than older children or adults; and they spend more time indoors. Which of the following approaches should be considered in reducing indoor air pollutants?

a. Eliminating or controlling the sources of pollution
b. Ventilating with outdoor air to dilute and remove pollutants
c. Air cleaning by air filters and ionizers to remove some airborne particles
d. a and b only
e. All of the above

110. An estimated 4,000 toxic substances have been isolated in cigarette smoke. Some of these substances are clearly termed toxic, and others carcinogens. Which of the following substances in cigarette smoke has (have) been categorized as carcinogenic?

a. Benzo-*a*-pyrene
b. *N*-Nitrosodimethylamine
c. Cadmium
d. a and c only
e. All of the above

111. A number of epidemiological studies have found a significant association between cancer and domestic exposure to pesticides. Evidence is increasing but still limited because of the methodological weaknesses of the research. Considering pediatric and adult malignancies, which of the following malignancies is (are) associated with exposure to pesticides?

a. Brain tumor
b. Prostate cancer
c. Non-Hodgkin lymphoma
d. a and c only
e. All of the above

112. Prenatal and postnatal effects of environmental tobacco smoke predispose to several health conditions. You are an environmental health educator in a high-risk environment for tobacco, and you are required to address the health consequences of tobacco smoke. Which of the following conditions should be considered in your address?

a. Sudden infant death syndrome
b. Asthma
c. Ear infection
d. a and b only
e. All of the above

113. Occupational exposure to mercury is not uncommon. A survey conducted by the National Institute for Occupational Safety and Health (NIOSH) estimated that 70,000 American workers may be exposed to mercury vapors on the job. The result of this study is more likely to associate which of these professions with mercury exposure?

a. Laboratory technicians
b. Plumbers
c. Dentist and dental hygienists
d. Miners
e. All of the above

114. Dichlorodiphenyltrichloroethane (DDT) exposure has been related to the disruption of the endocrine and immune systems in humans. Reproductive or immune systems disruption may be caused by which of the following pesticides?

a. 1,2-dibromo-3-chloropane (DBCP)
b. Malathion
c. Parathion
d. Carbofuran
e. All of the above

115. The average amount of whole-body radiation exposure for an individual in the United States from all sources is estimated to be approximately 3.6 mSV (360 mrem) a year, or 0.01 mSv (1 mrem) per day. Because humans and other mammals are more sensitive to ionizing radiation relative to lower animals, higher doses of ionizing radiation may cause which of the following health effects in humans?

a. Mutations
b. Birth defects
c. Leukemia
d. Infertility
e. All of the above

116. The rising level of atmospheric carbon dioxide is indicative of global warming, which includes diminished crop yields, loss of biodiversity, rising sea levels, and environmental health problems as possible effects. The rate of global warming is due in part to increasing use of coal, oil, and gas to power the world's factories and vehicles. The widespread destruction of natural vegetation, particularly deforestation, contributes substantially to CO_2 emissions. As an environmental health specialist, which of the following policies should be considered important in reducing greenhouse gas emission, thus minimizing global warming?

a. Improving energy efficiency
b. Replacing fossil fuels with "soft energy path" technologies—switching to solar, wind, or wave power to generate electricity
c. Reversing forest loss
d. Reducing chloroflurocarbons
e. Taxing the use of fossils fuels
f. All of the above

117. There are several sources of water pollution with point sources and nonpoint sources as the two broad categories. The sources of water pollution include agriculture, construction activities, urban street runoff, and fallout of airborne pollutants. In the underdeveloped countries, contamination of waterways with microbial pathogens from human body waste remains a major public health problem. Which of the following pathogens is (are) associated with diarrheal illness caused by sewage-tainted drinking water?

a. Vibrio cholera
b. Shigella
c. Salmonella
d. E. Coli
e. Rotavirus
f. Girada Lamblia
g. All of the above

118. The Environmental Protection Agency estimates that the United States currently generates more than 300 million metric tons of industrial hazardous wastes annually. The mismanagement of these wastes can adversely affect human health and reduce the quality of life. What are the threats posed by careless disposal of these wastes?

a. Skin irritation and acute poisoning through direct contact
b. Fire and/or explosions
c. Air pollution
d. Surface water contamination
e. Groundwater contamination
f. All of the above

119. Polychlorinated biphenyls (PCBs) are primarily employed as cooling liquids in electrical transformers and capacitors. The U.S. Environmental Protection Agency estimates that 91% of all Americans have detectable levels of PCBs in their fatty tissues. Also, PCBs are associated with several health effects. Which of the following is (are) the adverse effects of PCBs?

a. Acne-like skin disorders
b. Burning sensation in eyes, nose, and throat
c. Hepatic dysfunction
d. All of the above
e. None of the above

120. Dioxin is chemically related to PCBs and other chlorinated hydrocarbons. All of the following are correct about this substance, *except*:

a. Dioxin produces chloracne in rabbits
b. Adverse effects in humans include immune system dysfunction
c. Fetal toxicity is observed in humans
d. None of the above
e. All of the above

121. Environmental agents such as cigarette smoke, radon gas, sunlight, heavy metals, X-rays, and chemical pesticides are known to be carcinogenic and are believed to be human carcinogens. The exact mechanisms by which these substances induce tumors are not fully understood, but are thought to involve multiple steps. Which of the following statements is (are) accurate concerning the steps in tumor induction?

a. Initiation is the first step and involves a change in the genetic material
b. The second step involves a process by which the initiated cells are exposed to another group of agents, termed promoters
c. Environmental carcinogens can bind to DNA nucleotides, thus forming DNA-carcinogenic adducts, leading to genetic damage and abnormal cellular proliferation
d. All of the above
e. None of the above

122. The growing recognition of the extent of lead contamination in U.S. housing prompted the federal government to take action in October 1995 and demand the disclosure of lead hazards in pre-1978 housing in any real estate transaction. The need for this action is due to the environmental health impact of lead associated with house paint. Which of the following adverse effects of lead has (have) been reported in the United States among children?

- **a.** High affinity for nerve tissue and hence neurotoxicity
- **b.** High blood lead level resulting in impaired intellectual ability in children
- **c.** Both of the above
- **d.** Neither of the above

123. Epidemiology could be defined as the study of distribution, determinants, and control of health-related states or events in the specified population and the application of this study to control health problems. As an epidemiologist, if required to fulfill the "distribution" and "determinant" components of this definition, what will this entail?

- **a.** Public health infrastructure
- **b.** Information, behavior, and health skills development
- **c.** Information dissemination to the population at risk
- **d.** Frequency, patterns, and causes of health-related events
- **e.** Prevention of health-related events

124. In a survey conducted to examine the prevalence of two diseases, *X* and *Y* in a specific population, the investigators found that the prevalence of disease *X* was higher than the prevalence of disease *Y*. If the incidence and seasonal pattern of both diseases are similar, which of these statements is (are) consistent with this observation?

a. Patients die quickly from disease *Y* but not disease *X*
b. Patients die quickly from disease *X* but not disease *Y*
c. Patients recover more quickly from disease *Y* than from disease *X*
d. Patients recover more quickly from disease *X* than from disease *Y*
e. a and c only

125. The approach to epidemiology can be described as descriptive, which involves the analysis of disease, disabilities, and injury patterns by person, place, and time. During summer 2006, there was an outbreak of bacterial meningitis in Nocity, Illinois. If you are appointed to investigate this epidemic using descriptive epidemiologic approach, what are the main reasons for describing this outbreak by person, place, and time?

a. To assess the health status of the Nocity population
b. To generate a hypothesis about the causal factors (causative pathogens) for this epidemic
c. To plan and evaluate the public health programs to manage this epidemic
d. a and c only
e. All of the above

126. During the third week of January 2006, 80 persons of a total population of 450 in Newtown attended a wedding ceremony, which included a meal prepared by several of the participants. Within 2 days, 35 of the participants became ill with salmonellosis. Estimate the attack rate among the participants.

a. 7.7/100
b. 43.7/100
c. 17.7/100
d. 21.2/100
e. None of the above

127. In a small community of 1,000 households with a population of 5,000 people, 150 persons were affected with E. Coli gastroenteritis in 100 households. A total of 500 persons lived in the 100 affected households. If each household had only one primary case, estimate the secondary attack rate.

a. 12.5%
b. 30.0%
c. 10.0%
d. 25.0%
e. 37.5%

128. The following table shows the number of persons who ate egg salad and those who did not and those who developed group A streptococci and those who did not. Using this information, estimate the relative risk of Group A streptococci in the exposed.

Exposure	Group A Streptococci	Non-Group A Streptococci	Total
Egg salad	46	22	68
Non-egg salad	13	46	59
Total	59	68	127

a. 0.68
b. 3.07
c. 0.22
d. 7.39
e. 0.88

129. In the Framingham Heart Study (FHS), the residents of the state of Massachusetts have been followed since the1950s to identify occurrence (heart disease) and risk factors for heart disease. This study identified high blood pressure, hyperlipidemia, stress, and physical inactivity as risk factors in heart disease. This dynamic cohort now involves the grandchildren of the original cohort. Which of the following study designs represent this study?

a. Case-crossover
b. Ambi-directional cohort
c. Retrospective cohort
d. Case-control
e. None of the above

130. A study was conducted in which men (15–49 years) with testicular neoplasm and a comparable group of men (15–49 years) without testicular neoplasm were asked about their prior use of steroidal anti-inflammatory drugs. If you assume that the subjects were selected on the basis of disease and not exposure, and the risk as a measure of association is not directly estimated but obtained as odds ratio, this is an example of which type of design(s)?

a. Experimental
b. Observational
c. Cohort
d. Case-control
e. b and d only

131. Epidemiologic designs are largely observational. Often, the critical issue restricting the conduct of experimental, clinical, or intervention trial is the ethical consideration such as assigning humans to a known carcinogen such as nicotine. Which of the following statements illustrate the distinction between the two designs?

a. Investigator is "blinded" (prevented from knowing the subject's true exposure status until the end of the study) in an experimental study but not in an observational study
b. Investigator controls the subject's outcome in an experimental study but not in an observational study
c. Investigator controls the subject's exposure in an experimental study but not in an observational study
d. Experimental studies are conducted with animals; observational studies are conducted with humans
e. a and c only

132. Confounding is the mixing effect of an extraneous variable in the association between the predictor (independent variable) and outcome (dependent variable). A study was conducted to examine the association between pancreatic cancer and coffee drinking. If a third variable, cigarette smoking, is assumed to be a confounder in this association, which of the following features will qualify smoking as a confounder in this association?

a. Smoking is associated with coffee drinking in the population that produced the cases
b. Smoking is an independent cause or predictor of pancreatic cancer
c. Smoking is not an intermediate step in the causal pathway between coffee drinking and pancreatic cancer
d. a and c only
e. All of the above

133. Which of the following statements is *incorrect* regarding public health?

a. The focus of a public health intervention is to prevent rather than treat a disease through surveillance of cases and the promotion of healthy behaviors
b. Public health is fulfilling society's interest in ensuring conditions in which people can be healthy
c. Immunization programs and distribution of condoms are examples of public health measures to control disease at the population level
d. Public health is concerned with medical care rather than preventive services
e. Public health focuses on prevention research rather than biomedical research

134. Which of the following statements is *inaccurate* regarding the history of public health?

a. The miasmatic theory of disease held that disease such as cholera or the Black Death was caused by "bad air"
b. Robert Koch postulated the germ theory of disease
c. John Snow, following the cholera epidemic in Central London in 1854, disproved the miasmatic theory of disease causation
d. Edward Jenner utilized vaccination in the 1880s to treat smallpox
e. Jonas Salk developed the Hepatitis B vaccine to prevent viral hepatitis infection in the United States in 1955

135. A 45-year-old Hispanic-American woman residing in San Antonio, Texas, has a history of breast cancer in her family. On a visit to her primary care physician, she is scheduled to undergo both breast and cervical cancer screening. These services are considered to be:

a. Primary prevention
b. Secondary prevention
c. Tertiary prevention
d. Routine medical examination
e. None of the above

136. The Boston City Health Department plans to reduce exposure to cigarettes in order to decrease the incidence of bladder cancer among its residents by implementing tobacco education sessions at all schools in the city. This approach best describes:

a. Health promotion
b. Disease prevention
c. Disease screening
d. All of the above
e. None of the above

137. The Centers for Disease Control and Prevention (CDC) assessed the rate of dental caries among inner-city African-American children in Baltimore, Maryland, and recommended water fluorination. This approach is best described as:

a. Health promotion
b. Disease prevention
c. Disease screening
d. a and c only
e. None of the above

138. The San Francisco City Health Department decides to immunize all high school students against Hepatitis B, which denotes an action, logically taken, to prevent the development of Hepatitis B infection in this group of school children who are well and do not have Hepatitis B viral infection. This approach to disease prevention constitutes an example of:

a. Tertiary prevention
b. Disease screening
c. Secondary prevention
d. Primary prevention
e. Disease prognosis
f. None of the above

139. Assessment and policy development in public health require an understanding of the causes of health problems at the population level and depend on the knowledge provided by biomedical sciences, social and behavioral sciences, and environmental sciences. Which of the following sciences of public health is (are) the basis for the assessment function of public health?

a. Management and policy science
b. Epidemiology
c. Public health biology
d. Biostatistics
e. b and d only
f. None of the above

140. Public health focus is on preventive measures, which makes its goal more abstract than medicine, rendering its achievement more difficult to recognize. As a public health professional, which of the following statements could *most appropriately* define your function?

a. Disease prevention and control
b. Disease identification
c. Health promotions
d. All of the above
e. None of the above

141. The graduate students at the Tulane University School of Public Health and Tropical Medicine are required by the Louisiana State Department of Health to determine the rate of prostate cancer among African-American males in the state. Which of the following is (are) needed to achieve this public health core function of assessment?

a. Data collection
b. Data analysis and interpretation
c. Communication of information for action or intervention
d. a and b only
e. All of the above

142. The U.S. Department of Health and Human Services, through the Centers for Disease Control and Prevention, has proposed the role of public health in disaster preparedness such as Hurricane Katrina. Which of these is *not* the direct function of public health in disaster preparedness?

a. Prevention of disaster
b. Coordinating the response to disaster
c. Reducing the rate of causality through careful and strategic planning to treat the affected persons
d. Minimizing further casualties
e. None of the above

143. Global warming or climate change reflects the modern challenge to public health initiative in preventing diseases and promoting the health of the population. There are logical and practical health concerns as the consequence of global warming. Which of the following conditions should be considered as the effect of such a climate change?

a. Emerging hyperthermia and heat stroke
b. Increase in cardiovascular diseases especially among the vulnerable populations
c. Increase in pulmonary disorders such as asthma
d. All of the above
e. None of the above

144. The Healthy People 2010 objectives call on public health to reduce health disparities. As a public health professional entrusted with the responsibility of reducing health disparities in breast cancer, which of the following areas of disparities should be an important step in arriving at this goal?

a. Education
b. Race/ethnicity
c. Income
d. Age
e. All of the above

145. Public health achievements are often unrecognized. If you are elected as the director of a state health department and you are requested to convince the elected officials of the achievements of public health during the 21st century in this nation, which of the following should you consider as part of the top 10 accomplishments of public health?

a. Routine use of vaccination and healthier mothers and babies
b. Improvement in motor vehicle safety and fluoridation of water

c. Safer workplaces and safer and healthier foods
d. Control of infectious disease and decline in deaths from heart disease and stroke
e. b and c only
f. All of the above

146. As a newly assigned director of the county's health department, you are required to brief the commissioner's court on the challenges of public health in your county in order to prepare a long-term budget to address these issues. Given the general knowledge of what public health will be facing in the future, which of the following areas should you include in your briefing?

a. Emerging infectious disease such as AIDS/TB, antibiotics resistance, and foodborne pathogens
b. Aging and the related chronic disabilities and chronic diseases
c. Obesity and overweight and its consequences
d. Disaster and bioterrorism preparedness
e. b and c only
f. All of the above

147. You are recently appointed to direct the chronic disease prevention program for the elderly in the state of Illinois, and your goal at interview was morbidity compression. Which of the following interventions should be considered beneficial in your program?

a. Smoking cessation
b. Dietary modification
c. Physical activities
d. Recreational activities
e. a and c only
f. All of the above

148. The population mean visit to a public health clinic is 5 patients per day, and the standard error is 0.5 visits. Calculate the 95% confidence interval, given that the *z*-score for this confidence limit is 1.96.

a. ± 0.98
b. ± 0.5
c. ± 0.82
d. ± 1.29
e. None of the above

149. If 50% (0.5) of the population received immunization against flu virus during the winter season, 2006, and the standard error from this proportion is 2.5% (0.025), what is the 90% confidence interval, given that the *Z*-score is 1.645?

a. ± 2.5%
b. ± 4.1%
c. ± 6.4%
d. ± 4.9%

150. The scale of measurement is essential in the planning of an analysis of public health data. The presence of prostate cancer is measured in binary scale, whereas smoking status (none, light, moderate, and heavy) is measured in ordinal (categorical) scale. Which of the following scales will be an adequate measure for diabetes death rate (deaths per 100,000 persons)?

a. Binary
b. Continuous
c. Ordinal
d. Nominal
e. None of the above

151. Which of the following data will have a normal distribution shape?

a. Annual income in the year prior to starting graduate school in 2006
b. Number of hours of health events watched last week by a random sample of public health nurses
c. Blood pressure in the population of all African-American women
d. Hospital length of stay in days for 989 randomly selected patients for a community hospital
e. None of the above

152. A small mean difference in a paired *t*-test produces a small *p* value if the sample size, *n*, is large. Which of the following statements support this observation?

a. The larger the sample size, the smaller the standard error of the mean
b. The standard error is the denominator in the test statistic, and a smaller denominator produces a larger test statistic
c. The larger the test statistic, the smaller the *p* value
d. The smaller the test statistic, the smaller the *p* value.
e. a, b, and c only

153. Which of the following is (are) accurate concerning analysis of variance (ANOVA)?

a. It compares means across more than two independent groups
b. It tests the null hypothesis that all population means are equal versus the alternate hypothesis that at least one population group means is different from others
c. If null is rejected, multiple two sample *t*-test must be performed to determine which mean(s) is (are) different
d. It can be used to assess whether or not mean lycopene serum level differs among Caucasian, African-American, and Asian men
e. All of the above

154. The following table shows an output of an analysis conducted to assess the relationship between needle sharing and tuberculosis among 268 intravenous drug users. One hundred and two of the participants admitted to sharing needles. Of these 102, 27 tested positive with a tuberculin test. The other 166 subjects denied having shared needles, and of these 166, 30 had a positive tuberculin test.

	Exposed	Unexposed	Total
Cases	27	30	57
Noncases	75	136	211
Total	102	166	268
Risk	0.2647059	0.1807229	0.2126866
Point estimate	[95% Confidence Interval]		
Risk difference	0.083983	−0.0197312	0.1876972
Risk ratio	1.464706	0.9267407	2.314955
Attributable. fraction. sample	0.3172691	−0.0790505	0.5680262
Attributable. fraction. population	0.1502854		
chi2(1) = 2.66 Pr > chi2 = 0.1028			

From this output, which of the following statements is (are) appropriate?

a. There is a statistically significant risk difference for tuberculosis comparing needle sharers and nonsharers
b. Needle sharers are statistically significantly greater than 2 times more likely to be tested positive for tuberculosis with tuberculin test
c. There is a nonstatistically significant increased risk of tuberculosis among needle sharers relative to those who do not share needles in this sample of intravenous users
d. a and c only
e. None of the above

155. The quality of a sampling estimate could be measured by random error. Random error refers to:

a. Precision and validity
b. Lack of precision
c. Precision but lack of validity
d. None of the above
e. All of the above

156. Which of the following is (are) examples of nonprobability samples?

a. Convenience samples
b. Snowball sampling
c. Purposive sampling
d. All of the above
e. None of the above

157. Which of the following is (are) *accurate* concerning probability sampling?

a. Each subject has a known probability of being selected
b. It allows the application of statistical sampling theory to hypothesis testing and generalization
c. Both of the above
d. Neither of the above

158. Which of the following is (are) *true* concerning simple random sampling?

a. There is an equal chance of drawing each unit
b. It requires listing of all sampling units in the sampling frame
c. It requires numbering of all units and random draw of units
d. Sampling error is easily measured
e. All of the above

159. Which of the following is (are) *true* regarding systematic sampling?

a. Requires selection of sample at regular intervals based on sampling fraction
b. Requires complete list of sampling units from the sampling frame
c. Simple to perform, and sampling error is easily measured
d. Disadvantages include periodicity
e. All of the above

160. As a newly hired public health analyst, you are required to obtain a sample of 90 children from the Well Child Program for a study to assess the effect of vitamin supplements on childhood growth. There are 1,800 children in the sampling frame. All of the following will be accurate regarding your approach, *except*:

a. The sampling fraction = 20
b. Sampling frame list subjects from 1 to 1,800
c. A number between 1 and 20 is randomly selected
d. If the first person selected is 10th in the sampling frame, the second person will be the 32nd
e. If the first person selected is 8th in the sampling frame, the second person to be selected is the 28th

161. Sample size estimation prior to the conduct of study is necessary to reliably measure factor of interest and detect significant association. Often, there is a trade-off between the study size and resources. Which of the following factors is (are) needed for sample size estimation?

a. Significance level (alpha)
b. Power (1-beta)
c. Expected prevalence of the factor of interest
d. a and c only
e. All of the above

162. You are involved in a descriptive survey to examine the association between physical activities and overweight and obesity. If the sampling technique in the study involves simple random or systematic sampling, absolute or desired precision is 0.03, the prevalence of physical activity is 15%, and alpha risk expressed in *Z*-score is 1.96, what will be an estimated sample size for this study?

a. 1,088
b. 544
c. 833
d. 163
e. None of the above

163. Which of the following considerations is (are) necessary if you are expected to estimate the sample size needed to examine, using a case-control design, the association between testicular neoplasm and HIV infection among African-American males?

a. Odds ratio worth detecting
b. Proportion of exposed persons in the source population
c. Desired level of significance (α)
d. Power of the study ($1 - \beta$)
e. All of the above

164. The prevalence of the factor of interest in the population is 70%, and the desired precision is 0.05. The alpha risk expressed as *Z*-score is 1.96. Estimate the sample size needed in each group for the comparison of two proportions/groups.

a. 707
b. 1,414
c. 24
d. 324
e. None of the above

165. Which of the following is (are) *accurate* regarding the power of a statistical test?

a. Probability that the test will reject a false null hypothesis
b. Probability that a study will not result in type II error
c. The higher the power, the greater the chance of obtaining a statistically significant result when the null hypothesis is false
d. Statistical power depends on significance criterion as well as the effect size or the size of the difference
e. All of the above

166. The following table presents the STATA output of the mean baseline and 6 months' follow-up of systolic blood pressure of African-American men ($n = 10$), aged 35 to 48 treated with daily beta blocker and a diuretic. Which of the following statements is (are) accurate?

Paired *t*-Test

Variable	Obs	Mean	Std. Err.	Std. Dev.	[95% Conf.	Interval]
Baseline	10	124	3.42215	10.82179	116.2586	131.7414
Follow-up	10	112.6	2.62128	8.289217	106.6703	118.5297
Difference	10	11.4	1.681269	5.316641	7.596704	15.2033

Mean(diff) = Mean(Baseline − Follow-up)	$t = 6.7806$	
Ho: mean(diff) = 0	Degrees of freedom = 9	
Ha: Mean(diff) < 0	Ha: Mean(diff) != 0	Ha: Mean(diff) > 0
$Pr(T < t) = 1.0000$	$Pr(\|T\| > \|t\|) = 0.0001$	$Pr(T > t) = 0.0000$

a. The use of beta blocker and diuretic in these men with hypertension is associated with the decrease in the mean systolic blood pressure in this sample
b. The paired *t*-test tests the null hypothesis that that the two population means are not equal
c. Assumes that the paired scores of the subjects are normally distributed
d. a and c only
e. None of the above

167. Understanding what *p* means requires understanding the logic of statistical hypothesis testing. For example, suppose an investigator wants to test whether or not Tamoxifen decreases breast cancer recurrence. He or she will select two groups of women diagnosed and treated for breast-localized breast cancer through surgery and administer Tamoxifen to one group and placebo to the other. The odds ratio of breast cancer recurrence will be obtained, comparing the two groups. To determine if the observed odds ratio is not due to random variation, an arbitrary cutoff point, termed a significance level, of 0.05 is often selected and termed *p* value. Which of the following statements is (are) *true* concerning the interpretation of the *p* value?

a. The probability of the sample data arising by chance
b. The probability of obtaining a value of the test statistic as large as or larger than the one computed from the data when in reality there is no difference between the different treatment groups
c. The probability of being wrong when asserting that a true difference exists between the two treatment groups
d. The chance of getting the observed effect if the null hypothesis was false
e. b and c only

168. An investigation was conducted to examine the relationship between serum cholesterol and BMI measured in kg/m^2. The study was analyzed using the correlation coefficient technique as the purpose of the design was not to use BMI to predict serum cholesterol level. Which of the following statements is (are) *true* regarding this statistical method?

a. Only provides evidence of the causal relationship between two variables
b. Is inappropriate when there is an underlying relationship between the two variables, but it is not linear
c. Should only be used to judge the biological importance of the two variables
d. Should not be performed unless the two variables are measured on continuous scale and are both normally distributed
e. If the correlation is greater than zero (0), then serum cholesterol and BMI are said to be positively correlated

169. A study was performed to determine neonatal weight (g) from maternal preconception weight (kg). A random sample of 100 mothers and their newborn babies ($n = 100$) were weighed. Which of the following statements is (are) accurate regarding the interpretation or the statistical technique for the analysis of this study?

a. A two-sample *t*-test is adequate
b. Conditional logistic regression is appropriate
c. Simple linear regression can be used to describe the straight line relationship between maternal preconception weight and neonatal weight
d. Neonatal weight (Y) can be predicted from maternal preconception weight (X)
e. c and d only

170. Most public health data involve the presence or absence of disease, termed binary outcome. The logistic regression model is an adequate predictive model in examining the association between an explanatory or independent variable measured in continuous, categorical, or binary scale. Which of the following is (are) correct regarding the statistical model underlying the logistic regression model?

a. $\ln(P/1 - P) = \beta_0 + \beta_1 X_1$
b. $Y = \beta_0 + \beta_1 X_1$
c. $\ln(P/1 - P) =$ log odds (or logit) of disease risk
d. $\beta_0 =$ log odds ratio associated with X_1 (exposure)
e. a and c only

171. The scale of variables is important in the selection of statistical methods. Which of the following statements is (are) accurate concerning dependent/response or outcome variable in linear and logistic models?

a. Outcome is continuous in logistic model
b. Mean μ of outcome Y, $-\infty < \mu < +\infty$ in linear model
c. Outcome is categorical in linear model
d. $P = \Pr(\text{disease}) = \text{logit}(P) = \ln(p/1 - p)$ in logistic model
e. b and d only

172. African-American race/ethnicity is a known risk factor for hypertension. A study was conducted to determine the association between hypertension and salt intake in a sample of 250 White and 250 Black males. The investigators utilized the logistic regression model for their analysis in order to generate the coefficients (β) to relate hypertension to salt intake (X_1) and hypertension to race (X_2). What is the accurate interpretation of β_1?

a. Log odds of hypertension among the unexposed
b. Log odds of hypertension associated with salt intake
c. Change in the mean hypertension with a unit change in salt intake given that race is held at constant
d. Log odds of hypertension associated with race
e. None of the above

173. Low birth weight is an outcome that is a public health concern, because infant mortality rates and birth defects are higher for low-birth-weight babies. Maternal behavior during gestation is a predisposing factor in pregnancy outcomes. As a public health statistician, if you are investigating the association between preconception obesity and low birth weight, and if there are age-matched controls (non-obese mothers), which of the following statistical techniques will be most adequate in the analysis of your data if the outcome (low birth weight) is binomial?

a. Unconditional logistic regression
b. Conditional logistic regression
c. Simple linear regression
d. Multiple linear regression
e. None of the above

174. A study was conducted to determine an association between daily exercise and colorectal cancer. The result indicated a relative risk of 0.8 and a 95% confidence interval, 0.7–1.3 for daily exercise relative to nondaily exercise in developing colorectal cancer over 10 years. The authors claimed that daily exercisers have a relative risk of 0.9 compared to nondaily exercisers in developing colorectal cancer over 10 years. Which of the following statements is correct regarding this finding?

a. The study had sufficient power to detect a true difference if one existed
b. The authors should have reported a 90% confidence interval
c. The authors are 95% confident that the null hypothesis is true
d. Type I error could have occurred
e. None of the above

175. A public health scientist wanted to calculate the linear association between low-density lipoprotein (LDL) and prostate-specific antigen. The two variables are continuous, but the joint distribution is not Gaussian. Which of the following statistical methods may be *most* appropriate?

a. Simple linear regression
b. Spearman correlation coefficient
c. Pearson's correlation coefficient
d. Cox proportional hazards model
e. Poisson regression

176. A nutrition questionnaire was administered by e-mail to 837 U.S. male physicians on two separate occasions, 6 months apart. The questions to which responses were requested included the quantities of food eaten for 125 separate food items. The following table displays the data obtained from the two surveys on the amount of fish consumed. Which of the following test statistics will produce the quantitative measure of reproducibility between the responses of the two surveys?

Amount of Fish Consumption Reported by 837 U.S. Male Physicians in Two Different Surveys

	Survey 1 ≤1 Serving/Day	Survey 2 > 1 Serving/Day	Total
≤1 serving/day	236	142	378
> 1 serving/day	119	340	459
Total	355	482	837

a. Chi square statistic
b. Kappa statistic
c. Specificity
d. Spearman's correlation
e. Sensitivity

Questions 177–179 (*fictitious data*). Investigators conducted a study to evaluate the use of magnetic resonance imaging (MRI) in the diagnosis of brain attack. One hundred and sixty patients with brain attack confirmed by surgery were evaluated with MRI, as were 100 patients without brain attack. The MRI results were positive in 112 patients with brain attack and in 20 of the patients without the condition.

177. What is the false-positive rate in this study?

a. 30%
b. 20%
c. 70%
d. 80%
e. 85%

178. What is the likelihood ratio positive of this test?

a. 0.2
b. 0.7
c. 3.5
d. 0.28
e. None of the above

179. What are the chances of having brain attack if the MRI is positive? Calculate the positive predictive value based on the given data.

a. 0.85 (85%)
b. 0.15 (15%)
c. 0.18 (18%)
d. 0.70 (70%)
e. None of the above

180. Which of the following statistical methods will be adequate to test the null hypothesis that maternal serum testosterone level, which is a postulated risk factor in testicular neoplasm, does not differ among African-American and Caucasian women, given that testosterone is measured in an interval scale and is normally distributed in these populations?

a. Mann–Whitney rank-sum test
b. Chi-square statistic
c. Unpaired *t*-test
d. Friedman statistic
e. Wilcoxon signed-rank test

181. In a study conducted to examine the correlation between alcohol consumption and systolic blood pressure in a sub-population of U.S. males, the investigators reported a significant positive correlation between these two variables. From this correlation, we may conclude that:

a. Subjects who consume less alcohol are at lower risk of increased systolic pressure
b. High alcohol consumption can cause increased systolic pressure
c. Subjects who consume less alcohol are at higher risk of increased systolic pressure
d. No association exists between alcohol consumption and systolic pressure
e. Low alcohol consumption can cause increased systolic pressure

182. Using statistical thinking to reach conclusions in epidemiologic and biomedical research amounts to much more than memorizing a few formulas and looking for *p* values in the tables. Applying statistical techniques and the results require insights into the scientific hypothesis. All of the following should be clearly stated by the investigator regarding the scientific hypothesis, *except*:

a. The name of the funding agency for the research and the affiliation of the principal investigator (PI) with the funding agency
b. The data used to test the hypothesis
c. The procedure used to collect the data
d. The population the samples represent
e. The statistical procedure used to evaluate the data and reach the conclusions

183. An epidemiologist wishes to study whether obesity is associated with prostate cancer. If in reality, the presence of obesity leads to prostate cancer with a relative risk of 3.0, the epidemiologist wants to have a 95% chance of detecting an effect this large in the planned study. This statement is an illustration specifying:

a. Statistical power
b. An odds ratio
c. Hazards ratio
d. Type I or alpha error
e. Type II or beta error

184. A biostatistician observed a relationship between two measures (amount of contaminated water with fecal contents and frequency of diarrhea) to be linear, and the coefficient of determination has a value near 1.0. A scatterplot of the observations will be a:

a. Horizontal straight line
b. Vertical straight line
c. Straight line that is neither horizontal nor vertical
d. Random scatter of points about the regression line
e. Positive slope

185. Holmes and colleagues (2007) conducted a study to determine the effectiveness of androgen deprivation therapy (ADT) on loco-regional prostate cancer. The authors reported that the effect of ADT on survival was assessed using Kaplan–Meier's method, log-rank test, and Cox proportional hazards. Which of the following statements is (are) true regarding the log-rank test in their analysis techniques?

a. Compares data on those who received ADT relative to those who did not
b. Tests the null hypothesis that each group (ADT and non-ADT) has the same force of mortality

c. Calculates the probability that the observed death would have occurred in the ADT group and the probability that it would have occurred in the non-ADT group
d. a and c only
e. All of the above

Questions 186–187. The accompanying table gives some of the results from the same study (Holmes et al., 2007). This table presents the multivariable result of the effect of ADT on the overall survival of older men treated for loco-regional prostate cancer.

Effect of Androgen Deprivation Therapy on Overall Survival of Older Men Treated for Local/Regional Prostate Cancer in 1992–1999 SEER Areas

Hazard Ratio (95% Confidence Interval) of All-Cause Mortality in Cases Receiving ADT, Primary Therapy, and Chemotherapy

	Model I		Model II	
Covariates	**HR**	**95% CI**	**HR**	**95% CI**
Androgen deprivation therapy (ADT)				
No	1.0	Reference	1.0	Reference
Yes	1.29	1.24–1.34	1.04	1.00–1.08
Primary therapy (PT)				
WW	1.0	Reference	1.0	Reference
RP	0.20	0.19–0.21	0.32	0.30–0.33
XRT	0.47	0.45–0.48	0.63	0.61–0.65
RP/XRT	0.29	0.26–0.32	0.40	0.36–0.45
Chemotherapy				
No	1.0	Reference	1.0	Reference
Yes	0.93	0.90–0.98	1.01	0.97–1.05

Notes: Model I adjusted for primary therapy and chemotherapy. Model II adjusted for sociodemographics, comorbidity, tumor characteristics, and primary therapies plus chemotherapy. Abbreviations: watchful waiting (WW) or observational management, radical prostatectomy (RP), radiation therapy (XRT), hazard ratio (HR), and confidence interval (CI).

Source: Holmes, L., et al. Effectiveness of androgen deprivation therapy in prolonging survival of older men treated for loco-regional prostate cancer. *Prostate Cancer and Prostatic Diseases,* 2007, doi:10.1038/sj.pcan.4500973.

186. The hazard ratio for the effect of primary therapy (PT) on survival is presented with watchful waiting as the reference. What is the interpretation of the hazard ratio (HR) of 0.32 and 95% confidence interval 0.30–0.33 for the effect of radical prostatectomy (RP) on survival?

a. Surgery relative to watchful waiting or observational management significantly reduces the risk of dying by 68%
b. Surgery relative to watchful waiting or observational management significantly reduces the risk of dying by 32%
c. Watchful waiting relative to surgery increases the risk of dying by 32%
d. There is a statistically nonsignificant 32% increased risk of dying in subjects undergoing watchful waiting compared with subjects undergoing surgery
e. There is a statistically nonsignificant 68% decreased risk of dying in subjects undergoing surgery compared with subjects undergoing observational management or watchful waiting

187. Based on the information in the table, what conclusion could be draw from this study on the effect of ADT in prolonging survival of older men treated for loco-regional prostate cancer?

a. ADT significantly increases survival by 4%
b. There was a nonsignificant decrease in survival due to the use of ADT
c. ADT nonsignificantly decreased survival by 40%
d. There was an increased survival of 40% among the subjects who did not use ADT
e. None of the above

188. Which of the following is (are) method(s) of depicting frequency distribution?

a. Histograms
b. Stem leaf
c. Boxplots
d. Quantiles
e. All of the above

189. In an intervention program to control blood pressure among 36 inner-city African-American women aged 36 to 56 years, at the end of the intervention an investigator found the mean systolic blood pressure to be 123.1 mm/Hg and a standard deviation of 11.3 mm/Hg. If standard error (SE) is calculated, what will this be?

a. 1.88 mm/Hg
b. 2.02 mm/Hg
c. 10.89 mm/Hg
d. 3.42 mm/Hg
e. None of the above

190. A study examined glucose tolerance and insulin sensitivity in normal and overweight hyperthyroid inner-city Hispanic-American women. If the authors wanted to compare the baseline glucose (mg/dl) in the women to see if weight or thyroid level had an effect, which of the following statistical methods will be most appropriate?

a. Two-way ANOVA
b. One-way ANOVA
c. Logistic regression
d. Paired *t*-test
e. Correlation analysis

191. (Fictitious study) A study was designed to examine the relationship between children's age and daily consumption of apple and orange juices. There were 100 two-year-old children [$<$ 12 fluid ounces of juice/day (n) $=$ 75, and $\geq$ 12 fluid ounces/day (n) $=$ 25] and 85 five-year-old children [$<$ 12 fluid ounces of juice/day (n) $=$ 70, and $\geq$ 12 fluid ounces/day (n) $=$ 15]. The combined age (2 years and 5 years, n $=$ 185) indicated that $<$ 12 fluid ounces of juice/day (n) $=$ 155, and $\geq$ 12 fluid ounces/day (n) $=$ 30. What is the best statistical method to determine whether or not there is a difference between the 2-year-olds and 5-year-olds regarding the daily consumption of apple and orange juices?

a. Pearson correlation
b. Fishers exact test
c. Paired *t*-test
d. Fisher's *Z*-distribution
e. ANOVA

192. Chlamydia trachomatis (CT) is an established pathogenic microbe in non-gonococcal urethritis, pelvic inflammatory disease, and other infectious diseases. An investigator wishes to conduct a study to examine the risk factors associated with CT using 862 female undergraduate students. He or she intends to control for several risk factors simultaneously in the analysis of variables associated with CT. If CT is measured in binary scale, which of the following analytic methods might be appropriate?

a. Multivariate logistic regression
b. Multivariable logistic regression
c. Simple linear regression
d. Stratified analysis
e. Conditional multivariable logistic regression

193. An investigator wishes to examine the relation between cholesterol as a risk for heart disease. If he or she chooses to measure cholesterol using an interval scale, which of the following scales will be adequate in measuring heart disease (outcome variable)?

a. Binary
b. Ordinal
c. Interval
d. Continuous
e. Quantitative

194. Which of the following statements is (are) *accurate* concerning behavior change theory?

a. Purpose theory explains why the target of change is chosen
b. Explanatory theory discusses what modifiable factors contribute to the problem
c. Change theory explains the strategies that are employed to change the modifiable factors or behavior
d. a and c only
e. All of the above

195. Which of the following statements is (are) *correct* regarding the use of theory in behavior intervention?

a. Change theory is used to predict behavior change
b. Theories that match unit of practice appear to be most adequate in behavior change
c. Theories need to be made practical by developing programs that identify program objectives linked to causal relationships within theory
d. All of the above
e. None of the above

196. Social learning/cognitive theory had been employed in interventions to reduce HIV risky behaviors among the population at risk. Self-efficacy and response efficacy are observed to be associated with behavior expectation and outcome expectation, respectively. Which of the following statements *best* describe response efficacy in an intervention to increase condom use among high-risk youths?

a. Belief that specific action will influence condom use
b. Belief in skills and confidence to use condoms
c. Both of the above
d. Neither of the above

197. The marginalization model of disease and health status suggests integration and protective factors, namely, physical, economic, occupational, social, political, and cultural. Which of the following factors may be considered as host vulnerability in this model?

a. Genetic
b. Bio-behavioral
c. Psychosocial
d. Environmental
e. All of the above

198. Public health can be defined as what we as a community can do collectively to stay healthy. As a newly appointed health director of a county health department, which of the following should you attempt to put in place in order to fulfill this overall goal of public health in your county?

a. Improvement in the quality of life for all
b. Permitting and promoting healthy behaviors
c. Minimizing and eliminating health hazards
d. Protecting, preserving, and restoring the natural environment
e. All of the above

199. Risky behaviors are predisposing factors to cardiovascular diseases, teenage pregnancy, injuries, diabetes mellitus, and HIV infection. As a behavior interventionist for a city health department, which of the following risky behaviors should you address in order to reduce the incidence of these diseases or conditions?

- **a.** Physical inactivity
- **b.** Poor nutrition
- **c.** Early sexual activity and unprotected sex
- **d.** a and c only
- **e.** All of the above

200. Public health is influenced by multiple factors—mainly, politics, economics, environment, culture, ideology, and race/ethnicity. Multilevel intervention is considered the hallmark of intervention in changing behavior and promoting health. Which of the following levels should you include in your intervention if you are assigned to promote heart health by eliminating cigarette smoking?

- **a.** Individual
- **b.** Family and household
- **c.** Institutional and organizational
- **d.** Social and community network
- **e.** All of the above

ANNOTATED ANSWERS

1. The correct answer is **E** (core functions of public health).

2. The correct answer is **D** (core functions of public health).

3. The correct answer is **D** (core functions of public health).

4. The correct answer is **E** (public health achievement in the 21st century).

5. The correct answer is **E** (public health achievement in the 21st century).

6. The correct answer is **D** (public health focus).

7. The correct answer is **C** (study validity—bias). Because men with diabetes mellitus are monitored more than men who do not have DM, disease ascertainment may be better in the monitored population and may introduce surveillance bias (monitoring of one population [diseased] more than the other [disease-free]). This bias may lead to erroneous estimation of the effect of the disease in the monitored population, thus inflating the point estimate (RR, OR) (Gordis, *Epidemiology*, 3rd ed., 2004, p. 227).

8. The correct answer is **C** (study validity—confounding). In all subjects without stratification by BMI, there is a strong association between exercise and type II DM, with low exercise as a risk factor, RR = 4.2 (26.25 / 6.25), where 26.25 is the incidence in those with low exercise (105 / 4,000 × 1,000). The RR in those with BMI > 24.99 kg/m^2 = 3.0 (30 / 10) and that in BMI < 24.99 kg/m^2 = 3.0 (15 / 5). Regardless of BMI, the best estimate of the effect of exercise on type II DM is 3.0. The crude estimate of 4.2 is indicative of the confounding effect of BMI on the association between exercise and type II DM. Moreover, BMI itself is a risk for type II DM, as comparison here shows that low exercise subjects are much more obese in terms of their distribution by person-years: 75% versus 25% (high exercise).

9. The correct answer is **D** (study validity—confounding).

10. The correct answer is **A** (interaction). Assuming the additive model, the expected incidence rate for joint exposure to smoke and air pollution is 40 (baseline rate), which is the rate in those unexposed to neither of the two exposures + 360 (400 − 40), (which is the rate in those with smoke minus the

baseline rate) + 160 (200 − 40), which is the rate in those exposed to air pollution minus the baseline rate. Substituting in the additive model: 40 + 360 + 160 = 560 per 10,000 person-years. Therefore, the incidence rate in those with joint exposure is 560 per 10,000.

11. The correct answer is **C** (interaction). Assuming the joint multiplicative effect of the two exposures, the relative risk for smoking is, RR = 10 (400 / 40), where 40 is the baseline rate, the reference (1.0), and the relative risk for air pollution is RR = 5 (200 / 40), again where 40 is the baseline risk. The joint relative risk is 50 (10 × 5). The expected incidence rate for the joint exposure is then computed by multiplying the joint relative risk by the baseline rate. Substituting: 40 (baseline rate) × 50 (joint relative risk) = 2,000 per 10,000 person-years.

12. The correct answer is **D** (effect measure modifier). Because the difference between the crude OR (6.6) and the M-H adjusted OR by age (6.3) is less than the difference considered to be significant in establishing confounding (10.0%), age is not a confounding or there is very little confounding by age. In addition, the odds of smoking in the different age groups are very different, indicative of the role of age as effect measure modifier. Statistically, the presence of differences in the stratified OR (stratum-specific OR) is indicative of the possibility of interaction (effect measure modifier). Age therefore modifies the effect of smoking on cancer of the cervix in women (Gordis, *Epidemiology*, 3rd ed, 2004, pp. 233–234; Aschengrau & Seage, *Essentials of Epidemiology*, 2003, pp. 337–341).

13. The correct answer is **B** (study design). Randomization is one of the three main ways to control for confounding at the design phase of a study. This method, which is restricted to experimental design, ensures that the treatment assignment occurs in an unbiased manner, and results in the balanced distribution of known and unknown confounders (Aschengrau & Seage, *Essentials of Epidemiology*, 2003, p. 288).

14. The correct answer is **B** (case-control study). Case-control design is relatively inexpensive to conduct compared with prospective cohort design. In comparison to case-control, this is one of the disadvantages of prospective cohort studies.

15. The correct answer is **D**. The standardized mortality ratio is calculated by the formula: Observed death/Expected death. To obtain the expected number of deaths, the number of person-years from each age group is multiplied by the age-specific mortality rate in the standard population. The observed number of deaths is then divided by the sum of expected number of deaths. Substituting, Observed (12) / Expected (7.10) = 1.69.

Age Group	Number of Person-years (*P*)	Mortality Rate in Standard Population per 100,000 (*R*)	Expected Number of Deaths (R × P)
25–34	7,557	0.8	0.06
35–44	4,023	4.8	0.19
45–54	2,961	47.9	1.42
55–64	2,043	265.8	5.43
Total			7.10

16. The correct answer is **C** (case-control design).

17. The correct answer is **D** (ecologic design).

18. The correct answer is **E** (study validity). Epidemic study aims to establish association between risk factors, often called exposure or independent variables, and the outcome/response variable, which could be a disease, disability, or injury. The presence of an association may be the result of a factual relationship between these variables, which is broadly termed causal. For association to be causal, both bias and confounding must be eliminated as possible explanations of the association. In contrast, association may be noncausal or artifactual, implying that the finding is either influenced by bias or confounding (Aschengrau & Seage, *Essentials of Epidemiology*, 2003, pp. 251–252).

19. The correct answer is **D** (rates comparison). The crude mortality rates are inadequate in comparing the mortality events of two populations because populations differ with respect to age distributions and with advanced age associated with increasing mortality. Therefore, to adequately compare two populations in terms of mortality rates, age-adjusted rate is preferable, which removes the confounding or differences imposed by the differences in the age distribution of the population (Friis & Sellers, *Epidemiology for Public Health Practice*, 1996, pp. 91–92).

20. The correct answer is **A** (the relationship between incidence, prevalence, and disease duration). The prevalence of disease (assuming low prevalence) is associated with both incidence and the duration of the disease. The prevalence is the product of the incidence and the disease duration ($P = ID$), where P is the prevalence, I is the incidence of the disease, and D is the disease duration. The duration of the disease is influenced by (a) fatality or mortality or (b) prognosis (recovery). If the incidence of the disease is higher in one population (A) than the other population (B) and the prevalence is the same in both populations, the possible explanations are (a) the case fatality for the disease is higher in population A, or (b) the recovery is quicker in population A (Aschengrau & Seage, *Essentials of Epidemiology*, 2003, pp. 48–49).

21. The correct answer is **C** (measure of association in case-control study). The association between osteoporosis and low-calcium intake in this design (case-control) can be estimated with the odds ratio (measure of association in case-control), which is the odds of exposure in the disease divided by the odds of the exposure in the non disease. Using the 2 × 2 table, the odds ratio is mathematically given by AD/BC. Substituting, $(40 \times 80) / (60 \times 20) = 2.66$ (Garb, *Understanding Medical Research: A Practitioner's Guide*, 2000, pp. 33–35, 131–132).

22. The correct answer is **A** (measure of risk difference). The attributable benefit (same as attributable risk) is calculated by first calculating the mortality benefit in the exposed to the antiretroviral drug and the mortality benefit in those not exposed to the antiretroviral drug. The attributable benefit is the difference between the benefit in those exposed to the treatment and the benefit of those not exposed. Substituting, (a) Mortality rate in the exposed $= 4/55 \times 100 = 7.3\%$; (b) Mortality rate in the unexposed $= 14/52 \times 100 = 26.9\%$. The attributable benefit or risk is computed by mortality rate in the unexposed minus the mortality rate in the exposed. Substituting, $26.9\% - 7.3\% = 19.6\%$.

23. The correct answer is **E** (clinical trial).

24. The correct answer is **D** (clinical trial).

25. The correct answer is **C** (case-control).

26. The correct answer is **A** (epidemiologic causal inference).

27. The correct answer is **C** (bias).

28. The correct answer is **C** (criteria for confounding).

29. The correct answer is **E** (bias-systematic error).

30. The correct answer is **E** (sources of epidemiologic data).

31. The correct answer is **E** (cross-sectional design).

32. The correct answer is **B** (measure of disease occurrence).

33. The correct answer is **C** (internal validity).

34. The correct answer is **D** (measures of risk). *Absolute risk* is the outcome events divided by the population at risk. This measure identifies the actual events rate in the population in question. *Absolute risk increase* is the pre-intervention absolute risk minus the post-intervention absolute risk. This measure identifies the absolute increase in the rate of specific adverse events associated with an intervention. *Absolute risk reduction* is the pre-intervention absolute risk minus the post-intervention absolute risk. This measure identifies the absolute decrease in the rate of specific adverse events associated with the intervention. Attributable risk percent is the attributable risk divided by the risk in the exposed times 100. This measure expresses the degree to which risk for a specific outcome is due to a specific exposure. Attributable risk (AR) is computed by the risk in the exposed minus the risk in the unexposed, and it provides the measure of absolute risk associated with the exposure.

35. The correct answer is **B** (publication bias in meta-analytic design).

36. The correct answer is **A** (hazard ratio interpretation).

37. The correct answer is **E** (health policy and disease prevention).

38. The correct answer is **C** (health policy and the Congress).

39. The correct answer is **E** (health insurance dynamics).

40. The correct answer is **D** (health insurance eligibility).

41. The correct answer is **B** (private health insurance coverage).

42. The correct answer is **E** (racial health disparities elimination).

43. The correct answer is **E** (health disparities narrowing).

44. The correct answer is **E** (health insurance coverage).

45. The correct answer is **E** (enforcing laws and regulations regarding the health of the public).

46. The correct answer is **D** (strategies to improve insurance coverage). Other suggestions include (a) mandate businesses to offer coverage, (b) offer tax credits or other assistance to help purchase private coverage, and (c) expand Medicare to uninsured under 65 (Kaiser Family Foundation Health Poll Report, October 2007).

47. The correct answer is **E** (bio-psychosocial aspect of health and illness).

48. The correct answer is **E** (intervention model and risk reduction).

49. The correct answer is **D** (behavioral and psychosocial aspect of terrorism).

50. The correct answer is **E** (behavioral and social factors in health).

51. The correct answer is **E** (socioeconomic and social class determinant of health).

52. The correct answer is **E** (smoking as a modifiable risk factor in disease causation and mortality).

53. The correct answer is **G** (ecologic model of health behavior).

54. The correct answer is **E** (psychosocial model of behavior).

55. The correct answer is **E** (influence of stress and social support on health behavior).

56. The correct answer is **E** (racial disparities in health).

57. The correct answer is **E** (social support system and health outcomes).

58. The correct answer is **D** (health belief model of behavior change).

59. The correct answer is **D** (research translation—efficacy to effectiveness).

60. The correct answer is **B** (behavioral intervention).

61. The correct answer is **D** (behavioral intervention).

62. The correct answer is **A** (behavioral intervention strategies).

63. The correct answer is **D** (population health determinants).

64. The correct answer is **E** (obesity epidemic and health consequences).

65. The correct answer is **E** (disease specific intervention).

66. The correct answer is **D** (socio-demographic influence on smoking).

67. The correct answer is **D** (influence of education on youth health-risk behavior).

68. The correct answer is **E** (health survey study—longitudinal design).

69. The correct answer is **C** (multiple regression analysis).

70. The correct answer is **C** (analysis of variance—ANOVA).

71. The correct answer is **E** (nonparametric analysis).

72. The correct answer is **D** (health behavior models).

73. The correct answer is **D** (health disparities).

74. The correct answer is **D** (government role/policy in health promotion).

75. The correct answer is **E** (racial variation in cause-specific infant mortality).

76. The correct answer is **C** (behavior change model).

77. The correct answer is **C** (teratogens).

78. The correct answer is **E** (transport pollutants).

79. The correct answer is **D** (EMF and childhood leukemia). In 2001, an expert scientific working group of WHO's International Agency for Research on Cancer (IARC) reviewed studies related to the carcinogenicity of static and extremely low frequency (ELF) electric and magnetic fields. Using the standard IARC classification that weighs human, animal, and laboratory evidence, ELF magnetic fields were classified as "possibly carcinogenic to humans" on the basis of epidemiological studies of childhood leukemia, which showed, on average, a twofold excess of leukemia associated with living near power lines. The IARC "strength of evidence" for this risk is halfway between the strongest categories ("a human carcinogen" or a "probable carcinogen") and the weakest ("insufficient evidence" and "probably not a carcinogen") in their 5 categories. It is possible that there are other explanations for the observed association between exposure to ELF and childhood leukemia, and the extent of the hazard, if true, appears to be small.

80. The correct answer is **D** (risk process).

81. The correct answer is **D** (risk process).

82. The correct answer is **C** (risk assessment). Human data are the most desirable to identify the primary hazard in the hazard identification step and are given highest priority because there may be species differences in toxic response.

83. The correct answer is **D** (risk assessment and structure-activity relationship).

84. The correct answer is **D** (possible human carcinogen). If sufficient evidence in animals (positive test results in more than one species or study), the substance can be considered as a possible human carcinogen. Inadequate evidence in humans means that no satisfactory epidemiology study exists.

85. The correct answer is **D** (toxic effect of substances and risk assessment). The primary toxic effect which determines the type of procedure to be used in conducting a risk assessment is evidence that the chemical is carcinogenic. The risk assessment for carcinogens is quite different from that of non-carcinogens. Carcinogenic effects are viewed as non-threshold effects and non-carcinogenic effects are considered to have dose thresholds.

86. The correct answer is **E** (environmental impact of pesticide use). Direct killing of organisms exposed to chemicals, indirect killing via depletion of food or habitat, groundwater contamination, and indirect contamination via food chains are all environmental impacts of pesticide use (Nadakavukaren, *Our Global Environment*, 1995, pp. 301–309).

87. The correct answer is **D** (environmental media prediction method). Because actual measurements of environmental chemical exposure are often unavailable, exposure models are used. Models can predict future movement into areas that are currently free from contamination.

88. The correct answer is **D** (exposure assessment).

89. The correct answer is **E** (exposure assessment).

90. The correct answer is **B** (exposure assessment). A major aspect of the exposure assessment is to identify the exposure pathways. Also, all potential exposure pathways are carefully considered as well as contaminant releases, movement, and fate in the environment and the exposed populations.

91. The correct answer is **E** (exposure pathways).

92. The correct answer is **C** (risk characterization). Risk characterization is the process in which the dose-response assessment and exposure assessment are integrated to predict risk to specific populations. It is the final stage in the risk assessment process and involves the prediction of the frequency and severity of effects in exposed populations.

93. The correct answer is **A** (cancer risk estimation). An increased cancer risk of 2.0×10^{-6} means that it is likely that 2 persons in 1 million will develop the specific type of cancer in their lifetime due to exposure to the chemical.

94. The correct answer is **E** (major outdoor air pollutants).

95. The correct answer is **E** (health effect of air pollutants).

96. The correct answer is **E** (health effects of secondhand tobacco smoke—air pollutant).

97. The correct answer is **D** (health effect of particulate matter).

98. The correct answer is **E** (sources of indoor air pollutants).

99. The correct answer is **D** (acute health consequences of indoor air pollutants).

100. The correct answer is **D** (chronic health effect of indoor air pollutants).

101. The correct answer is **E** (sources of carbon monoxide).

102. The correct answer is **E** (signs and symptoms of carbon monoxide poisoning).

103. The correct answer is **C** (primary prevention of CO poisoning).

104. The correct answer is **E** (secondhand smoking and children's health).

105. The correct answer is **E** (health effects of biologic pollutants).

106. The correct answer is **D** (aflatoxins and carcinogenicity).

107. The correct answer is **E** (Sick Building Syndrome).

108. The correct answer is **E** (radon migration system). www.epa.gov/iaq/radon/construc.html

109. The correct answer is **E** (indoor air quality). www.epa.gov/iedweb00/pubs/hpguide.html

110. The correct answer is **E** (carcinogens in tobacco smoke).

111. The correct answer is **E** (pesticides and human cancer).

112. The correct answer is **E** (environmental tobacco smoke and health consequences).

113. The correct answer is **E** (occupational exposure to mercury).

114. The correct answer is **E** (pesticides and immune and reproductive health effects) (Nadakavukaren, *Our Global Environment*, 1995, pp. 312–317).

115. The correct answer is **E** (ionizing radiation and human health) (Nadakavukaren, *Our Global Environment*, 1995, pp. 377–380).

116. The correct answer is **F** (control of global warming).

117. The correct answer is **G** (sewage-tainted drinking water and causative pathogens of diarrheal disease).

118. The correct answer is **F** (hazardous waste and environmental health).

119. The correct answer is **D** (toxic substances and health effect) (Nadakavukaren, *Our Global Environment*, 1995, pp. 241–243).

120. The correct answer is **D** (dioxin and health effect).

121. The correct answer is **D** (carcinogenesis). Initiation is the first step and involves a change in the genetic material. Environmental carcinogens can bind to DNA nucleotides, thus forming DNA-carcinogenic adducts, leading to genetic damage and abnormal cellular proliferation. The second step involves a process by which the initiated cells are exposed to another group of agents, termed promoters. Environmental agents play a role in carcinogenesis as initiators, promoters, or both (Nasca & Pastides, *Fundamentals of Cancer Epidemiology*, 2001, pp 60–61, 68–69).

122. The correct answer is **C** (environmental health effect of lead).

123. The answer correct is **D** (meaning of epidemiology). Epidemiology refers to the study of the frequency, patterns, causes, and control and prevention of diseases, disabilities, and injuries in the human population. There are two main aspects of epidemiology: (a) distribution—epidemiology evaluates the distribution of health states by age, gender, race, geography, time, and so forth, and (b) epidemiology seeks to examine the association and causal association between the exposure and the health related states or events (Last, *A Dictionary of Epidemiology*, 3rd ed., 1995; MacMahan & Trichopoulos, *Epidemiology, Principles & Methods*, 2nd ed., 1996, p. 1).

124. The correct answer is **E** (factors influencing the prevalence of disease). Prevalence proportion does not measure disease onset but the disease status. Whereas incidence is a measure of risk, prevalence is not because it does not take into account the duration of disease. But prevalence is related to the duration of the disease and incidence of disease. Prevalence = Incidence × Disease duration. The number of people living with a disease (prevalence) will be influenced by the rate at which a new disease develops as well as the rate at which it is eliminated through cure (prognosis) or death (mortality). Therefore, the prevalence will increase if incidence increases and if there is improvement in treatment but not cure, and it will decrease if there is dramatic cure (quick recovery) (Gordis, *Epidemiology*, 3rd ed., 2004, p. 40; Aschengrau & Seage, *Essentials of Epidemiology*, 2003, pp. 48–49).

125. The correct answer is **E** (descriptive epidemiology).

126. The correct answer is **B** (primary attack rate). Attack rate, which is really a proportion and not a rate, is useful for comparing the risk of disease in groups with different exposures. This measure is calculated as Number of people at risk in whom a certain illness develops/Total number of people at risk. Substituting, 35/80 × (multiplier) = 35/80 × 100 → 43.75 per 100 (Gordis, *Epidemiology*, 3rd ed., 2004, p. 25).

127. The correct answer is **A** (secondary attack rate). Secondary attack rate yields the index of the spread of a disease within a family, household, dormitory, dwelling unit, etc. This measure is estimated as Number of new cases in group − Initial case(s)/Number of susceptible persons in a group − Initial case(s). Substituting: 150 − 100 (each household had one primary case and there were 100 households)/500 − 100 (primary case) × 100 → 50/400 × 100 = 12.5% (Mausner & Kramer, *Epidemiology—An Introductory Text*, 2nd ed., 1985, pp. 280–281).

128. The correct answer is **B** (relative risk/risk ratio). This is the measure of the strength of relationship between exposure and disease. Mathematically, RR = Risk or rate in the exposed/Risk or rate in the unexposed. Substituting: (46/68)/(13/59) → 3.07, implying that those exposed to egg salad had three times increased risk of developing group A streptococci (Aschengrau &

Seage, *Essentials of Epidemiology*, 2003, pp. 67–68; Mausner & Kramer, *Epidemiology—An Introductory Text*, 2nd ed., 1985, p. 169).

129. The correct answer is **E** (study design). In general, a design that begins with exposure(s) of interest and disease-free subjects and is aimed to assess the outcome in future by following the subjects represents a prospective cohort study. This is not a clinical trial or broadly intervention design because the subjects of the Framingham Heart Study (FHS) were not assigned but observed. The time relation in a prospective cohort study is present and future (continuing). A case-crossover design uses the previous experience of the cases as a substitute for a control series to estimate the person-time distribution in the source population. Ambi-directional cohort is a design that is both retrospective and prospective in its observation of the outcome. Retrospective cohort (historical cohort studies) is a design in which the cohorts are identified from recorded information and the time during which they are at risk for disease occurred before the beginning of the study. Simply, retrospective study is conducted by defining the cohort and collecting information which applies to past time. Case-control is a design in which the groups of individuals are defined in terms of whether they have or have not already experienced the outcome under consideration, and the exposure is then measured (Elwood, *Critical Appraisal of Epidemiological Studies in Clinical Trials*, 2nd ed., 2003, pp. 14–35; Rothman, *Epidemiology, An Introduction*, 2002, p. 89).

130. The correct answer is **E** (study design). This is an observational design because it involves natural observation without assignment. Case-control is a design in which the outcome had already occurred prior to the commencement of study, and study participants were selected on the basis of the disease. The direct measure of risk is not possible in case-control study but estimated as odds ratio.

131. The correct answer is **E** (experimental/clinical trial). Experimental design if feasible is considered the gold standard compared with observational studies. The active manipulation or assignment of the treatment by the investigator is the hallmark that differentiates experimental designs from observational studies. Whereas not all experimental designs utilize blindness to minimize bias, blindness is not a feature of observational designs. Neither in observational design nor experimental ones are investigators required to manipulate the outcome. Experimental designs, like observational ones, are conducted in human as well as animal populations (Aschengrau & Seage, *Essentials of Epidemiology*, 2003, pp. 163–165).

132. The correct answer is **E** (internal validity of study). Confounding is derived from the Latin *confondere*, meaning "to pour together," and indicates the confusion of two supposedly causal variables so that part or all of the purported effect of one variable (exposure) is actually due to the other (confounder). Confounding variable is considered an extraneous variable because it competes with the independent variable in explaining the outcome. In a study conducted to assess whether exposure (*A*) causes disease (*B*), *C* is a confounding if (a) *C* (smoking) is associated with *A* (coffee drinking) in the population that produced the cases *B* (pancreatic cancer); (b) *C* (smoking) is an independent cause or predictor of *B* (pancreatic cancer); or (c) *C* (smoking) is not an intermediate step in the causal pathway between coffee drinking (*A*) and pancreatic cancer (*B*) (Hennekens & Buring, *Epidemiology in Medicine*, 1987, pp. 287–293; Gordis, *Epidemiology*, 3rd ed., 2004, pp. 228–229).

133. The correct answer is **D** (mission and goal of public health). Public health definition remains complex. Broadly, the Committee for the Study of the Future of Public Health defines the mission of public health as fulfilling society's interest in ensuring conditions in which people can be healthy. Public health is concerned with disease control and prevention at the population level and focuses on preventive research. In contrast, public health focuses on preventive services rather than medical care services (Institute of Medicine, *The Future of Public Health,* 1988, pp. 1–17).

134. The correct answer is **E** (history of public health). The history of public health reflects the notion of disease causation and the measures to prevent diseases at the population level. The miasmatic theory dominated public health for a long period and was disproved by the germ theory. Koch's postulate in the 1880s represented a great notion of disease causation for the germ theory. John Snow, respected as the father of epidemiology, attributed the cholera epidemic in London in 1854 to polluted water. Jonas Salk in 1955 discovered the polio vaccine, which resulted in a remarkable reduction of polio cases in the United States (Institute of Medicine, *The Future of Public Health*, 1988, pp. 56–71).

135. The correct answer is **B** (methods of prevention). Preventing the occurrence of an illness, disability, or injury in the first place, by avoiding the risk or predisposing factors, refers to primary prevention. This denotes an action such as immunization taken to prevent the development of a vaccine-preventable disease in a person without the disease in question. The objective of secondary prevention is to minimize the severity of illness or damage to an injury-causing event once the event has occurred. Also, secondary prevention is aimed at early detection of a disease, either through screening or case finding, followed by treatment or intervention (e.g., the routine testing of stool for occult blood to detect treatable colon cancer in the early stage of the natural history of the disease). Tertiary prevention is aimed at medical treatment and rehabilitation as in stroke, with the intent to restore, improve, and prevent further neurological damage to the individual. Disease screening involves the identification of a subgroup of people who are at risk for having asymptomatic disease or who have a risk factor that predisposes them to developing a disease or becoming injured (Gordis, *Epidemiology*, 3rd ed., 2004, pp. 5–6).

136. The correct answer is **A** (behavioral intervention and health promotion). Health promotion is an intervention that seeks to eliminate or minimize risk exposure by modifying behavior, thus improving and protecting health.

137. The correct answer is **B** (intervention and disease control). Disease prevention is any intervention that is aimed at reducing or minimizing diagnosable conditions, such as immunization, water chlorination, and fluorination.

138. The correct answer is **D** (methods of prevention). *Primary prevention* denotes an action taken to prevent the development of a disease in a person who is well and does not have the disease in question. *Disease screening* is an action to identify those who are diseased, given the manifestation, and those who are not, given the absence of the manifestation. *Secondary prevention* denotes the identification of persons who have already developed Hepatitis B, for instance, at an early stage of Hepatitis B, through screening and early intervention. Identification of cases at an early stage in the natural history of the disease is indicative of the effectiveness of the intervention. *Disease prognosis* refers to the outcome of treatment following the diagnosis of the disease. *Tertiary prevention* involves treatment after disease (e.g., stroke) had been diagnosed and rehabilitation to prevent further health consequences (Schneider, *Introduction to Public Health*, 2nd ed., 2006, p. 12).

139. The correct answer is **E** (basic sciences of public health). *Epidemiology and biostatistics or biometry* are the basis of the assessment function of public health. Whereas epidemiology is involved in the design of study to assess the risk variable or determinants, statistics is essential in testing the hypothesis for possible inference, and statistical analysis is an integral part of an epidemiologic design. *Management and policy science* provide the basis for service provision and the evaluation of the public health programs, as well as the assurance that services are being provided and utilized by the population. *Pubic health biology* provides the information for the understanding of the disease or disabilities under assessment (Schneider, *Introduction to Public Health*, 2nd ed., 2006, pp. 8–9; Institute of Medicine, *The Future of Public Health*, 1988, p. 88).

140. The correct answer is **D** (core functions of public health). The Institute of Medicine describes the substance of public health as that of disease prevention and health promotion. The assessment function of public health denotes disease identification at the population level. All these represent the functions that are carried out by public health professionals in attempting to quantify disease, injury, or disability at the population level (Institute of Medicine, *Healthy Communities*, 1996, p. 8).

141. The correct answer is **E** (core functions of public health). The assessment function of public health calls for epidemiologic surveillance, which involves continuous data collection, analysis, interpretation, and information dissemination prior to intervention (Institute of Medicine, *The Future of Public Health*, 1988, pp. 1–17).

142. The correct answer is **A** (future and challenges of public health). Public health is challenged with increasing episodes of natural disasters, which are obvious threats to population health. The aftermath of hurricanes such as Katrina very clearly illustrate the deficiencies in the public health response to natural disaster. To prevent disaster is not a direct function of public health. Public health is charged with the coordination of an effective response in minimizing further causalities and improving the health of the survivors and preventing further causalities through collective and shared responsibilities of other governmental and private sectors (Schneider, *Introduction to Public Health*, 2nd ed., 2006, pp. 535–550).

143. The correct answer is **D** (public health and global warming). There is an association between seasonal variation and human health, including mental health. Extreme temperatures can result in failure in the thermoregulatory center, the hypothalamus, leading to death. Hospital data on admission on mortality indicate an increasing rate of death during extremely hot days especially among the elderly, young children, and those with chronic diseases. Also, extreme temperature can lead to increases in air and water pollution and the subsequent infectious diseases such as West Nile virus, cholera, and Lyme disease (pathogens affiliated with high heat as seen in summer). The physical effect of climate change is the alteration in the air temperature, thus increasing the concentration of ozone at ground level. Exposure to ozone, especially by those with already compromised cardiorespiratory function, may result in chest pain and pulmonary congestion (U.S. Global Change Research Program, *A Report of the National Assessment Synthesis Team, Climate Change Impacts on the United States—The Potential Consequences of Climate Variability and Change* http://www.usgcrp.gov/usgcrp/naac, accessed November 12, 2007).

144. The correct answer is **E** (health disparities and challenges of public health). The burden of disease is disproportionately shared in the United States as well as in other nations, including the United Kingdom. In the United Kingdom, where social class is obvious, the laborers are disproportionately affected compared with professional classes such as physicians and lawyers. In the United States, where social class remains an unpopular notion in research settings, socioeconomic variance is used to describe health disparities, with the economically marginalized, which implies the ethnic minorities (mainly African Americans), associated with the greatest burden of disease. Health disparity is also affected by education, age, and gender. In the United States, the observed racial/ethnic disparities in health are realistically driven by socioeconomic variance (Centers for Disease Control and Prevention, Eliminating Racial & Ethnic Health Disparities, http://www.cdc.gov/omhd, accessed November 15, 2007).

145. The correct answer is **F** (public health accomplishments). The CDC noted the top 10 accomplishments of public health during the 21st century as (a) routine use of vaccination, (b) healthier mothers and babies, (c) improvement in motor vehicle safety, (d) fluoridation of water, (e) safer workplaces, (f) safer and healthier foods, (g) control of infectious disease, (h) decline in deaths from heart disease and stroke, (i) access to family planning and contraceptive services, and (j) recognition of tobacco use as a health hazard. Remarkably, the increase in life expectancy has been associated with these achievements, mainly, the decline in deaths due to heart disease and stroke as a result of tobacco education and lifestyle modification in this direction (CDC, *MMWR*, 1999; 48:241–243).

146. The correct answer is **F** (challenges of public health). All are 21st-century public health challenges. Public health is threatened with the emerging infections and the antibiotic resistance associated with the changes in the envelope proteins of these pathogens as they continue to mutate. The epidemic of obesity and overweight presents a great challenge to public health and requires research and behavioral interventions in addressing its behavioral and lifestyle components. Realistically, the life expectancy gained by this nation in the areas of heart disease and stroke as a result of tobacco cessation and lifestyle modification in this direction will be lost to the obesity epidemic. Public health agencies need to act now in reducing the epidemic of obesity and overweight. Aging is not a pathologic process but is associated with the decline in biologic systems. To address successful aging, public health needs to prevent chronic diseases and chronic disabilities in the first place and compress morbidity. Therefore, to achieve successful aging or disease-free longevity is a challenge to public health in any society with an increase in the aging population. The increasing disparities in health, with the racial/ethnic minorities (mainly African Americans) being disproportionately burdened, is indicative of equitable provision of public health services to such vulnerable populations. Public health is challenged with confronting health with politics and allocating resources to those who cannot afford health care in our society (American Public Health Association 132nd Annual Meeting, November 6–10, 2004, Washington DC: Riscia, Prevention of Overweight and Obesity: Focus on Children and Adolescents; Ory, Emerging Issues in Geriatric Care: Aging and Public Health Perspectives; Glik, Bioterrorism Preparedness: Workforce, Organizational, Resources, and Risk Communication Issues).

147. The correct answer is **F** (chronic disease and challenges of public health). Morbidity compression refers to the delaying of illness (chronic diseases and disabilities) into oldest old age, with instant mortality at age 90 to 100 years.

Whereas aging is not a pathologic process, it is associated with decline in biologic functions, which could be delayed or improved by adequate lifestyle and health surveillance such as routine screening. An effective chronic disease program will benefit substantially from a well-designed intervention addressing cigarette and excessive alcohol consumption; dietary modification, with emphasis on a low-fat diet and increase in vegetables and fruits consumption; as well as 30 to 60 minutes of moderate exercise daily, because what matters for the aging biologic system is not the intensity of the exercise but the frequency for the reconditioning of the cardio-circulatory system and the musculature (American Public Health Association 132nd Annual Meeting, November 6–10, 2004, Washington DC: Ory, Emerging Issues in Geriatric Care: Aging and Public Health Perspectives).

148. The correct answer is **A** (confidence interval estimation from mean). The 95% CI is estimated by multiplying the standard error (SE) by the *Z*-score, which is 1.96. Using the formula and substituting: $0.5 \times 1.96 = 0.98$. Thus the lower confidence limit is $5 - 0.98 = 4.02$, while the upper confidence limit is $5 + 0.98 = 5.98$. The 95% CI = 4.02–5.98.

149. The correct answer is **B** (confidence interval estimation from proportion). Whether proportion or mean, 95% CI for a parameter is calculated by (Sample statistic) ±*(Standard error of sample statistic).

150. The correct answer is **B** (continuous measure).

151. The correct answer is **C** (normal distribution). Annual income in the year prior to starting graduate school in 2006 may be a skewed distribution. Number of hours of health events watched last week by a random sample of public health nurses may be bimodal, given different modes for male and female nurses. Blood pressure in the population of all African-American women in the United States may be a normal distribution. Hospital length of stay in days for 989 randomly selected patients for a community hospital may be skewed.

152. The correct answer is **E** (interpretation of paired *t*-test).

153. The correct answer is **E** (ANOVA).

154. The correct answer is **C** (interpretation of cross-sectional and cohort design analysis). The 95% CI for the risk ratio includes 1.0 (null), indicative of a non-statistically significant association. In addition, the *p* value for the chi-square is indicative of nonsignificant association at $\alpha < 0.05$ significance level.

155. The correct answer is **B** (random error as measure of precision).

156. The correct answer is **D** (sampling techniques).

157. The correct answer is **C** (probability sampling).

158. The correct answer is **E** (simple random sampling technique).

159. The correct answer is **E** (systematic sampling technique).

160. The correct answer is **D** (systematic sampling technique).

161. The correct answer is **E** (sample size estimation).

162. The correct answer is **B** (sample size estimation for descriptive survey). Using the formula for one proportion, $n = z^2 \times p \times q/d^2$, where n is the sample size, z is the alpha risk expressed in Z-score, p = the expected prevalence and $q = 1 - p$, and d is the absolute precision. Substituting, $1.96^2 \times 0.15 \times 0.85/0.03^2 = 544$.

163. The correct answer is **E** (sample size estimation for case control study). It is also essential to consider the number of controls per case.

164. The correct answer is **A** (sample size estimation—two proportions or groups). Using the formula, $n = z_1 - \alpha/2\ [P_1 (1 - P_1) + P_2(1 - P_2)]/d^2$, where n = sample size (each group), $z_1 - \alpha/2$ = confidence interval, P_1 = estimated proportion (larger), P_2 = estimated proportion (smaller), and d = desired precision. Substituting: $1.96^2\ [(0.70)(0.30) + (0.50)(0.50)]/0.05^2 = 707$.

165. The correct answer is **E** (statistical power of a test).

166. The correct answer is **D** (assumption and interpretation of paired or dependent *t*-test). The paired *t*-test tests the null hypothesis of no difference or equality of the two means (baseline relative to follow-up). Because the difference is greater than 0, the use of these two anti-hypertensive agents is associated with decrease in mean systolic blood pressure in this sample. Secondly, given the significance level, $p < 0.05$.

167. The correct answer is **E** (*p* value interpretation).

168. The correct answer is **E** (correlation coefficient).

169. The correct answer is **E** (simple linear regression).

170. The correct answer is **E** (logistic regression model).

171. The correct answer is **E** (characteristics of dependent variable in logistic and linear regression models).

172. The correct answer is **B** (interpretation of coefficient in logistic model).

173. The correct answer is **B** (analysis technique in matched-case control studies).

174. The correct answer is **D** (interpretation of 95% confidence interval).

175. The correct answer is **B** (nonparametric correlation regression).

176. The correct answer is **B** (reproducibility test). Reliability studies are designed to quantify the reproducibility of the same variable (e.g., daily dietary intake of a particular food), measured more than once. Kappa, which is a measure of agreement "beyond chance," is used as a measure of reproducibility between repeated assessments of the same variable. The chi-square test of association between the two surveys' responses, although performable, will not give a quantitative measure of the reproducibility between the responses on the two surveys. Using Kappa statistics (κ) is the appropriate test to measure reproducibility: $P_o - P_e / 1 - P_e$, where P_o is the observed probability of the concordance between two surveys, and P_e is the expected probability of concordance between the two surveys. Kappa is interpreted as, $\kappa > 0.75$ (75%) indicates excellent reproducibility, 0.4 (40%) $\leq \kappa \leq$ 0.75 (75%), good reproducibility while $0 \leq \kappa < 0.4$ (40%) denotes marginal/poor reproducibility. Also, +1.0 is indicative of a perfect agreement, while 0.0 indicates a complete independent between the two surveys. Specificity and sensitivity would be more appropriate indices of reliability or reproducibility if the investigators were interested in the concordance between responses on two different variables, where one of the variables is considered to be the gold standard (Abrahamson, *Making Sense of Data*, 2nd ed., 1994, pp. 171–182).

177. The correct answer is **B** (diagnosis and screening test). False-positive error rate (alpha error rate or type I error rate), simply refers to error committed by asserting that a proposition is *true*, when it is indeed *not true (false)*. If a test is not *specific*, this will lead to the test to falsely indicate the presence of a disease in nondisease subjects (cell B; see accompanying table). The rate upon which this occurs is termed false-positive error rate and is mathematically given by $B/(B + D)$. False-positive error rate is related to specificity: FP(rate) + Specificity = 1.0 (100%).

Test Result	Brain Attack Present	Brain Attack Absent	Total
Positive MRI	*A* (112)	*B* (20)	132
Negative MRI serving/day	*C* (48)	*D* (80)	128
Total	$A + C = (160)$	$B + D = (100)$	$(a + b + c + d) = 260$

Using the 2 × 2 contingent table, false-positive error rate = B/(B + D). Substituting: 20/100 = 0.2 (20%).

178. The correct answer is **C** (likelihood ratio of screening test). The likelihood ratio positive illustrates the ratio of sensitivity of a test ($a/a + c$) to the false-positive error rate ($b/b + d$) of the test. Using the formula, $a/(a + c) / b(b + d)$, substituting: 0.7/0.2 = 3.5.

179. The correct answer is **A** (positive predictive value). The positive predictive value (PPV) answers the question: If the patient's test result is positive, what is the probability that he or she has the disease? PPV indicates the proportion of the subjects who had positive MRI and had brain attack. Using the formula, PPV = $A / (A + B)$; substituting, 112 / (112 + 20) = 0.85 (85%).

180. The correct answer is **C** (hypothesis testing and statistic). An unpaired *t*-test is appropriate in testing the hypothesis comparing two groups that consist of different individuals, and the measurement scale is interval and drawn from normally distributed populations.

181. The correct answer is **B** (interpretation of correlation analysis). Correlation analysis is conducted to determine whether or not there is a relationship or an association. A significant positive correlation suggests that the relationship is directly proportional, meaning that *Y* (response variable—systolic pressure) increases as *X* (independent variable—alcohol consumption) increases.

182. The correct answer is **A** (scientific hypothesis testing).

183. The correct answer is **A** (statistical power).

184. The correct answer is **C** (graphic presentation of data).

185. The correct answer is **E** (test of significance for differences in survival). Success or effectiveness of treatment is measured in terms of time that some desirable outcome is maintained. Such analysis (time-related patterns of survival) yields survival analysis techniques that originated from the life table procedures. Kaplan–Meier also termed the product limit method that is more commonly used in biomedical and public health research compared to actuarial method. Kaplan–Meier's product limit and actuarial methods are commonly used methods to estimate survival experience of samples. Both methods are similar except that time since entry in the study is not divided into intervals for analysis in Kaplan–Meier product limit method.

Two or more life table curves could be tested to determine if they are significantly different. The *Z*-test for proportion is used for the actuarial curves, while the log-rank test is used for Kaplan–Meier curves. The log-rank test is an approximate chi-square test and compares the number of observed deaths in each group with the number of deaths that would be expected from the number of deaths in the combined groups, implying group membership or distinction did not matter. The log-rank test is also referred to as the Cox–Mantel log-rank statistic or Mantel log-rank statistic. The log-rank test, as may be incorrectly interpreted, does not involve ranking nor does it employ logarithm in its computation of the survival differences (Holmes et al., Effectiveness of Androgen Deprivation Therapy in Prolonging Survival of Older Men Treated for Loco-Regional Prostate Cancer, *Prostate Cancer and Prostatic Diseases;* doi:10.1038/sj.pcan.4500973).

186. The correct answer is **A** (interpretation of hazard ratio in Cox proportional hazard model).

187. The correct answer is **E** (hazards ratio and 95% confidence interval interpretation).

188. The correct answer is **E** (methods used in illustrating frequency distribution).

189. The correct answer is **A** (calculation of the standard error). The standard error allows the investigator to estimate the probable amount of error of the quantitative assertions, as well as enables the performance of statistical significance test (95% confidence interval). The standard error is calculated using the formula: $SE = SD/\sqrt{n}$, where n is the number of observations. Substituting: 11.3/6 = 1.88 mm/Hg. Please note that the larger the sample size (n), the smaller the standard error and the better the estimate of the population mean will be. Because SE can be converted to SD and vice versa, SD and SE are both acceptable measures of the amount of errors around the quantitative assertions.

190. The correct answer is **A** (two-way analysis of variance).

191. The correct answer is **B** (Fisher's exact test). When one or more of the expected, not the observed, counts in a 2×2 table is small (< 2), the chi-square test cannot be used; instead, the exact probability of finding the observed numbers by using Fisher's exact probability test is employed.

192. The correct answer is **B** (analysis of binary outcome data with several independent variables on mixed scales, controlling simultaneously for other variables).

193. The correct answer is **A** (scale of measurement of variables).

194. The correct answer is **E** (behavior change theories).

195. The correct answer is **D** (uses of theory in behavior intervention).

196. The correct answer is **A** (response efficacy).

197. The correct answer is **E** (marginalization model of disease/health status).

198. The correct answer is **E** (goal of public health and public health services in controlling diseases and promoting health).

199. The correct answer is **E** (behavioral risk factors and health outcomes).

200. The correct answer is **E** (public health causation theory and multilevel intervention). In addition to factors listed in the question, other levels to be considered in intervention are (a) living, working, and material conditions, and (b) local and national policies.

REFERENCES

Abrahamson, J. H. *Making Sense of Data*, 2nd ed. New York: Oxford University Press, 1994.

Ajzen, I. M. Prediction of Goal-Directed Behavior: Attitudes, Intentions, and Perceived Behavioral control. *Journal of Experimental Social Psychology* 22:453–474 (1986).

Aschengrau, A., & Seage III, G. R. *Essentials of Epidemiology.* Sudbury, MA: Jones & Bartlett, 2003.

Bandura, A. Perceived self-efficacy in the exercise of control over AIDS infection. In Mays, V. M., Albee, G. W., & Schneider, S. S. (Eds.), *Primary Prevention of AIDS: Psychological Approaches* (pp. 128–141). Newbury Park, CA: Sage, 1989.

Bhopal, R. Is Research into Ethnicity and Health, Racist, Unsound or Important Science? *BMJ* 314:1751–1756 (1997).

Briggs, D. Environmental Pollution and the Global Burden of Disease. *Br Med Bull* 68:1 (2003).

Centers for Disease Control and Prevention. Achievements in Public Health, 1900–1999: Changes in the Public Health System. *MMWR* 48(50):1141–1147 (1998).

Centers for Disease Control and Prevention. Annual Smoking-attributable Mortality, Years of Potential Life Lost, and Economic Costs—United States, 1995–1999. *MMWR* 51(14):300–303 (2002).

Centers for Disease Control and Prevention. Control of Infectious Diseases. *MMWR* 48:621–629 (1999).

Centers for Disease Control and Prevention. Decline in Deaths from Heart Disease and Stroke—United States, 1900–1999. *MMWR* 48:649–656 (1999).

Centers for Disease Control and Prevention. Eliminating Racial & Ethnic Health Disparities. Available at http://www.cdc.gov/omhd (accessed November 15, 2007).

Centers for Disease Control and Prevention. Family Planning. *MMWR* 48:1073–1080 (1999).

Centers for Disease Control and Prevention. Fluoridation of Drinking Water to Prevent Dental Caries. *MMWR* 48:933–940 (1999).

Centers for Disease Control and Prevention. Healthier Mothers and Babies. *MMWR* 48:849–857 (1999).

Centers for Disease Control and Prevention. Impact of Vaccines Universally Recommended for Children—United States, 1990–1998. *MMWR* 48:243–248 (1999).

Centers for Disease Control and Prevention. Improvements in Workplace Safety—United States, 1900–1999. *MMWR* 48:461–469 (1999).

Centers for Disease Control and Prevention. Motor-Vehicle Safety: A 20th Century Public Health Achievement. *MMWR* 48:369–374 (1999).

Centers for Disease Control and Prevention. Safer and Healthier Foods. *MMWR* 48:905–913 (1999).

Centers for Disease Control and Prevention. Ten Great Public Health Achievements in the United States, 1900–1999. *MMWR* 48:241–243 (1999).

Centers for Disease Control and Prevention. Tobacco Use—United States, 1900–1999. *MMWR* 48:986–993 (1999).

Committee on Assuring the Health of the Public in the 21st Century. *The Future of the Public's Health in the 21st Century*. Washington, DC: National Academy Press, 2002.

Crawford, B. L. Graduate Students in U.S. Schools of Public Health: Comparison of 3 Academic Years. *Public Health Rep* 94:67–72 (1979).

Dawson-Saunders, B., & Trap, R. G. *Basic and Clinical Biostatistics*, 2nd ed. Norwalk, CT: Appleton & Lange, 1994.

DiClemente, C., & Prochaska, J. O. Processes and stages of change: Coping and competence in smoking behavior change. In Shiffman, S., & Willis, T. A. (Eds.), *Coping and Substance Abuse* (pp. 319–334). San Diego, CA: Academic Press, 1985.

Elwood, M. *Critical Appraisal of Epidemiological Studies in Clinical Trials*, 2nd ed. New York: Oxford University Press, 2003.

Epidemiology Program Office, Office of the Director, CDC. Achievements in Public Health, 1900-1999: Changes in the Public Health System. *JAMA* 283:735–738 (2000). Available at http://jama.ama-assn.org/cgi/content/full/283/6/735 (accessed 3/5/2008).

Fishbein, M., & Ajzen, I. *Belief, Attitude, Intention, and Behavior: An Introduction to Theory and Research*, Reading, MA: Addison-Wesley,1975. Available at http://people.umass.edu/ajzen/f&a1975.html (accessed 12/12/2008).

Fishbein, M., Ajzen, I., & McArdle, J. Changing the behavior of alcoholics: Effects of persuasive communication. In Ajzen, I., & Fishbein, M. (Eds.), *Understanding Attitudes and Predicting Social Behavior*. Englewood Cliffs, NJ: Prentice-Hall, 1980.

Flies, J. L. *Statistical Methods for Rates and Proportions*, 2nd ed. New York: John Wiley & Sons, 1981.

Friis, R. H., & Sellers, T. A. *Epidemiology for Public Health Practice*. Frederick, MD: Aspen, 1996.

Garb, J. L. *Understanding Medical Research: A Practitioner's Guide*. Boston: Little, Brown, and Company, 2000.

Glik, D. C. Bioterrorism Preparedness: Workforce, Organizational, Resources, and Risk Communication Issues. Presented at American Public Health Association, 132nd Annual Meeting, November 6–10, 2004, Washington, D.C.

Gordis, L. *Epidemiology*, 3rd ed. Philadelphia: Elsevier Saunders, 2004.

Gordis L., et al. Privacy, Confidentiality, and Use of Medical Records in Research. *Science* 207:153–156 (1980).

Gordon, B., et al. *Inheriting the World, the Atlas on Children's Health and the Environment*. Geneva, Switzerland: World Health Organization, 2004.

Hennekens, C. H., & Buring, J. E. *Epidemiology in Medicine*. Boston: Little Brown & Company, 1987.

Hill, A. B. The Environment and Disease: Association or Causation? *Proc R Soc Med* 58:295–300 (1965).

Holmes, L., et al. Effectiveness of Androgen Deprivation Therapy in Prolonging Survival of Older Men Treated for Loco-regional Prostate Cancer. *Prostate Cancer and Prostatic Diseases*, doi:10.1038/sj.pcan.4500973, 2007.

Institute of Medicine. *Healthy Communities*. Washington, DC: National Academy Press, 1996.

Institute of Medicine. *The Future of Public Health*. Washington, DC: National Academy Press, 1988.

Jekel, J. F., Katz, D. L., & Elmore, J. G. *Epidemiology, Biostatistics, and Preventive Medicine*. Philadelphia: Saunders, 2001.

Kaiser Family Foundation Health Poll Report, *Kaiser Commission on Medicaid and the Uninsured*, October, 2007.

Katz, D. L. *Clinical Epidemiology & Evidence-Based Medicine: Fundamental Principles of Clinical Reasoning & Research*. Thousand Oaks, CA: Sage, 2001.

KKF/Harvard School of Public Health. *Health Care Agenda for the New Congress*, conducted November 4–28, 2004.

Last, J. M. *A Dictionary of Epidemiology*, 3rd ed. New York: Oxford University Press, 1995.

MacMachon, B., et al. Coffee and Cancer of Pancreas. *N Engl J Med* 304:630–633 (1981).

MacMahan, B., & Trichopoulos, D. *Epidemiology, Principles & Methods*, 2nd ed. Boston: Little, Brown, 1996.

Mausner, J., & Kramer, S. *Epidemiology—An Introductory Text*, 2nd ed. Philadelphia: Saunders, 1985.

Milbank Memorial Fund, The National Association of State Budget Officers, and the Reforming States Group, 2002–2003. State Health Expenditure Report, June 2005.

Mokdad, A. H., Marks, J. S., Stroup, D. F., & Gerberding, J. L. Actual causes of death in the United States. *JAMA* 291:1238–1245 (2000).

Molina, L. T. Megacities and Atmospheric Pollution. *J Air Waste Manag Assoc* 54:644 (2004).

Motulsky, H. *Intuitive Biostatistics*. New York: Oxford University Press, 1995.

Nadakavukaren, A. *Our Global Environment*. Long Grove, IL: Waveland Press, 1995.

Nasca, P. C., & Pastides, H. *Fundamentals of Cancer Epidemiology*. Frederick, MD: Aspen Publishers, 2001.

Ory, M. G. Emerging Issues in Geriatric Care: Aging and Public Health Perspectives. Presented at American Public Health Association, 132nd Annual Meeting, November 6–10, 2004, Washington DC.

Prochaska J. O., & DiClemente, C. C. Stages and processes of self-change of smoking: Toward an integrative model of change. *Journal of Consulting and Clinical Psychology* 51:390–395 (1983).

Prochaska, J. O., & DiClemente, C. *The Transtheoretical Approach: Crossing Traditional Boundaries of Therapy*. Homewood, IL: Dow Jones-Irwin, 1984.

Prochaska, J. O., DiClemente, C., & Norcross, J. In Search of How People Change: Applications to Addictive Behaviors. *American Psychologist* 47:1102–1114 (1992).

Prochaska, J. O., & Velicer, W. F. The transtheoretical model of health behavior change. *American Journal of Health Promotion* 12:38–48 (1997).

Riscia, P. M. Prevention of Overweight and Obesity: Focus on Children and Adolescents. Presented at American Public Health Association, 132nd Annual Meeting, November 6–10, 2004, Washington DC.

Roemer, M. I. Preparing Public Health Leaders for the 1990s. *Public Health Rep* 103:443–451 (1988).

Rothman, K. J. *Epidemiology, An Introduction*. New York: Oxford University Press, 2002.

Samet, J. M., et al. Epidemiology and Risk Assessment. *Am J Epidemiol* 148:929–936 (1998).

Schneider, M. *Introduction to Public Health*, 2nd ed. Sudbury, MA: Jones & Bartlett, 2006.

Scutchfield, D. F., & Keck, W. *Principles of Public Health Practice*, New York: Delmar Series in Health Services, 2002.

Senior, P. A., et al. Ethnicity as a Variable in Epidemiological Research. *BMJ* 309:327–330 (1994).

Soto, M. A., Abel, C., & Diever, A. (Eds). *Healthy Communities: New Partnership for the Future of Public Health*. Washington, DC: National Academy Press, Institute of Medicine, 1996.

Suk, W. A., et al. Environmental Threats to Children's Health in Southeast Asia and the Western Pacific. *Environmental Health Perspectives* 111:1340 (2003).

Taubes, G. Epidemiology Faces Its Limits. *Science* 269:164–169 (1995).

U.S. Department of Justice, Bureau of Justice Statistics. *State Prison Expenditures,* 2001. June 2004, NCJ 202949. Available at http://www.ojp.usdoj.gov/bjs/pubalp2.htm#spe (accessed 11/20/2007).

U.S. Environmental Protection Agency. *Indoor Air Pollution: An Introduction for Health Professionals.* Available at www.epa.gov (accessed November 12, 2007).

U.S. Global Change Research Program. *A Report of the National Assessment Synthesis Team, Climate Change Impacts on the United States—The Potential Consequences of Climate Variability and Change.* Available at http://www.usgcrp.gov/usgcrp/naac (accessed November 12, 2007).

Velicer, W. F., Norman, G. J., Fava, J. L., & Prochaska, J. O. Testing 40 predictions from the Transtheoretical Model. *Addictive Behaviors* 24:455–469 (1999).

Winkelstein, W., & French, F. E. The Training of Epidemiologists in Schools of Public Health in the United States: A Historical Note. *Int J Epidemiol* 2:415–416 (1973).

World Health Organization. *Development of WHO Guidelines for Indoor Air Quality. Report on a Working Group Meeting.* Bonn, Germany, October 23–24, 2006.

World Health Organization. *Establishing a Dialogue on Risks from Electromagnetic Fields.* Available at http://www.who.int/pehemf/publications/en/EMF_Risk_glossary_further.pdf (accessed November 12, 2007).

World Health Organization. *Radon and Cancer.* Available at http://www.who.int/mediacentre/factsheets/fs291/en/index.html (accessed October 29, 2007).

INDEX

C

D

E

F

G

H

I

J

K

L

M

Q

R

S

T

U

V

W

Z

p188 – Add to lecture 1 with answer